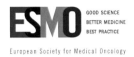

GOOD SCIENCE
BETTER MEDICINE
BEST PRACTICE

European Society for Medical Oncology

ESMO HANDBOOK OF
CANCER IN THE SENIOR PATIENT

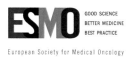

GOOD SCIENCE
BETTER MEDICINE
BEST PRACTICE

European Society for Medical Oncology

ESMO HANDBOOK OF
CANCER IN THE SENIOR PATIENT

Edited by

Dirk Schrijvers
Ziekenhuisnetwerk Antwerpen-Middelheim, Antwerp, Belgium

Matti Aapro
IMO Clinique de Genolier, Genolier, Switzerland

Branko Zakotnik
Institute of Oncology, Ljubljana, Slovenia

Riccardo Audisio
St Helens Teaching Hospital, St Helens, UK

Hendrik van Halteren
Ziekenhuis Gelderse Valle, Ede, The Netherlands

Arti Hurria
City of Hope, Duarte, California, USA

informa
healthcare

New York   London

Contents

Preface

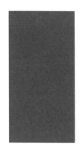

The European Society for Medical Oncology (ESMO) is to be complimented for having decided to dedicate an issue of its "Handbook" series to geriatric oncology. The International Society for Geriatric Oncology (SIOG) has been happy to help in the task of developing this volume, which was initiated by Dirk Schrijvers, Branko Zakotnik, Riccardo Audisio, Hendrik van Halteren, Arti Hurria, and the undersigned. This handbook is not only for Europeans. Cancer is a disease related to ageing, and the proportion of senior patients increases worldwide. While the proportion of persons beyond age 70 is still small in developing countries, their numerous population means that there are more "elderlies" in India than in Europe.

The authors have done a major effort in providing in record time chapters that truly reflect the state of the art in the management of senior adults with cancer. Many questions in this advancing field need considerable work before adequate guidelines can be provided. Nevertheless, progress is being made and is reflected by the contributions.

We recognize that some diseases have not been discussed and interesting topics have not been addressed. This gap is filled by more comprehensive books, and today's electronic communications allow one to explore any area of interest easily.

The treatment of any patient requires a careful evaluation of the person who is in need of such treatment. This is even truer for the seniors, who have less reserves to cope with cancer and its treatment. Therefore, this handbook leaves ample space for chapters that help in the delicate decision-making process, which should lead to the best therapy, adapted not only to the disease but also to the person who suffers from it.

Annals of Oncology, the official journal of ESMO, and the soon-to-be-launched Journal of Geriatric Oncology, official journal of SIOG, will keep us updated, as will all major medical journals. We know that this handbook, like any book, will need a second edition soon!

My last words go to Dirk, whose enthusiasm made this happen: thank you!

Matti Aapro
SIOG Executive Director

Contributors

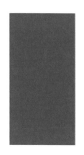

Amir E. Division of Hematology and Medical Oncology, Princess Margaret Hospital and University of Toronto, Toronto, Ontario, Canada

Audisio R.A. Department of Surgery, University of Liverpool, St Helens & Knowsley Teaching Hospitals, St Helens, Merseyside, U.K.

Balducci L. H. Lee Moffitt Cancer Center and Research Institute, Tampa, Florida, U.S.A.

Balk E.M. Department of Psychiatry and Behavioral Sciences, Memorial Sloan-Kettering Cancer Center, New York, New York, U.S.A.

Bellmunt J. Department of Medical Oncology, University Hospital del Mar-IMIM, Barcelona, Spain

Biganzoli L. Medical Oncology Unit, Hospital of Prato, Istituto Tumori Toscano, Prato, Italy

Campodonico F. Department of Urology, E.O. Ospedali Galliera, Genoa, Italy

Christoph D.C. Department of Medicine (Cancer Research), West German Cancer Centre, University Hospital of the University Duisburg-Essen, Essen, Germany

Coiffier B. Hospices civils de Lyon, Service d'Hématologie Clinique, Pierre Benite, France

Droz J.P. Department of Medical Oncology, Université de Lyon, Centre Léon Bérard, Lyon, France

Eberhardt W.E.E. Department of Medicine (Cancer Research), West German Cancer Centre, University Hospital of the University Duisburg-Essen, Essen, Germany

Extermann M. Moffitt Cancer Center, Tampa, Florida, U.S.A.

Fléchon A. Urologic Oncology Program, Department of Medical Oncology, Université de Lyon, Centre Léon Bérard, Lyon, France

Gaskell S. Mersey Deanery, Liverpool, Merseyside, U.K.

Gosney M. University of Reading, Reading, Berkshire, U.K.

Harrington K.J. The Royal Marsden Hospital NHS Foundation Trust, London, U.K.

Karapanagiotou E.M. Athens School of Medicine, Sotiria General Hospital, Athens, Greece; and The Royal Marsden Hospital NHS Foundation Trust, London, U.K.

Kristjansson S. R. Department of Geriatric Medicine, University of Oslo, Oslo University Hospital, Oslo, Norway

Maffezzini M. Department of Urology, E.O. Ospedali Galliera, Genoa, Italy

Michallet A.S. Hospices civils de Lyon, Service d'Hématologie Clinique, Pierre Benite, France

Nelson C.J. Department of Psychiatry and Behavioral Sciences, Memorial Sloan-Kettering Cancer Center, New York, New York, U.S.A.

Papamichael D. Department of Medical Oncology, B.O. Cyprus Oncology Centre, Nicosia, Cyprus

Roth A.J. Department of Psychiatry and Behavioral Sciences, Memorial Sloan-Kettering Cancer Center, New York, New York, U.S.A.

Schrijvers D. Department of Hemato-Oncology, Ziekenhuisnetwerk Antwerpen-Middelheim, Antwerp, Belgium

Seruga B. Division of Hematology and Medical Oncology, Princess Margaret Hospital and University of Toronto, Toronto, Ontario, Canada

Stauder R. Department of Internal Medicine V, Hematology and Oncology, Innsbruck Medical University, Innsbruck, Austria

Syrigos K.N. Athens School of Medicine, Sotiria General Hospital, Athens, Greece

Tannock I.F. Division of Hematology and Medical Oncology, Princess Margaret Hospital and University of Toronto, Toronto, Ontario, Canada

Terret C. PROLOG (Pilot Unit of Oncogeriatry in Lyon), Department of Medical Oncology, Université de Lyon, Centre Léon Bérard, Lyon, France

Tjalma W.A.A. Department of Gynaecological Oncology & University Multidisciplinary Breast Clinic Antwerpen, University Hospital Antwerpen, Antwerp (Edegem), Belgium

Weinberger M.I. Department of Psychiatry, Weill Cornell Medical College, White Plains, New York, U.S.A.

Wildiers H. Department of General Medical Oncology/Multidisciplinary Breast Centre, University Hospitals Leuven, Leuven, Belgium

Wolf D. Department of Internal Medicine V, Hematology and Oncology, Innsbruck Medical University, Innsbruck, Austria

Wyller T. B. Department of Geriatric Medicine, University of Oslo, Oslo University Hospital, Oslo, Norway

Zulian G.B. Department of Rehabilitation and Geriatrics, University Hospitals of Geneva, Geneva, Switzerland

Introduction

S. R. Kristjansson and T. B. Wyller
*Department of Geriatric Medicine, University of Oslo,
Oslo University Hospital, Oslo, Norway*

Defining the Elderly

There is no universally accepted age cutoff defining "elderly." This reflects the fact that chronological age itself is less important than biological events in driving the aging process within an individual. However, chronological age is a simple and practical way of defining a target population, and 70 years is the most commonly used cutoff for defining patients as elderly within the field of geriatric oncology.

Biology of Aging and Changes in Organ Function

Almost all age-related changes lead to reduced function. However, the elderly population is characterized by a marked variability in the rate of functional deterioration, both between individuals and within individuals. Three different trajectories of aging have been described.

- Aging with pathology and disability
- Normal aging with some disability
- Successful aging with minimal disability

The heterogeneity of the aging process has practical consequences for the assessment of elderly cancer patients: patients need individualized assessments to determine their *biological age*. Biological age is believed to reflect a person's remaining life expectancy and functional reserves. This will influence treatment decisions and predict treatment tolerance. There is no simple way to assess biological age, and the best tool available to date is a *comprehensive geriatric assessment* described in a separate chapter in this book.

Traditionally, within gerontology and geriatrics, natural age-dependent changes in structure or function of organs have been distinguished from age-related pathologies. This distinction is perhaps less useful from a practical point of view. Furthermore, normal age-dependent changes are believed to be associated with the prevalence of age-related pathologies, and disease in organs along with the aging process will exert synergistic effects on each other.

Another important characteristic of organ function and age is the close relation between supply and demand: cardiac output and respiratory function *at rest* remain largely unchanged with increasing age, but marked age effects appear when the systems need to perform under stress.

Within oncology, decreased organ function in the elderly may complicate treatment; impairments in renal, hepatic, and bone marrow function will increase drug toxicity. However, dose adjustments are usually not straight-forward because of the lack of accurate measurements of reserve capacity. Comorbidities may be associated with an increased risk of side effects and drug interactions. Again, because of the broad physiological variations seen among the elderly, valid generalizations are difficult to offer.

Changes in Cognition

Age is a risk factor for developing cognitive dysfunction. The prevalence of dementia in some studies is about 1% in 65- to 69-year-olds compared with 41% in those aged 90 and over. The presence of dementia or cognitive dysfunction seriously impacts cancer treatment. It is important to keep in mind that in some cases formal cognitive testing is the only way to identify cognitive dysfunction, especially if the patient has preserved language function or if the caregiver does most of the talking.

Pretreatment counseling often involves complicated decision-making weighing cost and benefit of different treatment options, and it is para-mount for the counseling physician to know whether the patient under-stands these issues.

For surgical procedures, the risk of postoperative acute confusional state (known as *delirium*) is markedly increased in the presence of preoperative cognitive dysfunction. Delirium can be prevented, as described below. When a patient is treated with chemotherapy, cognitive dysfunction raises issues regarding the patient's understanding of important signs of toxicity such as fever or bleeding, and arrangements of more intensive surveillance may be necessary. As both surgery under general anesthesia and chemotherapy treatment may alter cognitive function, it is important to consider whether the treatment places the patient at risk for being transferred from an independent to a dependent life situation.

Cancer and Aging

Increasing age is one of the strongest risk factors for cancer development. There is a marked increase in epithelial carcinomas from ages 40 to 80 years. Interestingly, beyond age 80 the incidence of cancers levels off. The link between cancer and aging is complex, and most of the fundamental questions still remain unanswered. In some instances, such as cellular senescence or telomere shortening, strategies that protect us from cancer may increase our rate of aging. However, cancer and aging also seem to share common etiologies such as genomic instability and reduced rate of autophagy.

We still do not know whether DNA damage is the ultimate stimulus to both cancer and aging. Another explanatory model views cancer and aging as stem cell diseases where cancer represents the effect of growth promoting mutations within a given stem cell, while aging represents the natural exhaustion and depletion of the stem and progenitor pool.

A common misconception among the general population as well as some doctors is that all cancers grow slowly in the elderly. This is true for some cancers, such as certain types of breast cancer and lung cancer, but the opposite is, for instance, true for acute leukemias, brain tumors, and ovarian cancer, which may be more aggressive in elderly patients.

Clinical Aspects

Because elderly patients often have reduced reserves in several organ systems, stress such as surgery, chemotherapy, or an acute infection may lead to general symptoms rather than organ-related symptoms. Thus, elderly patients often have occult or atypical presentations of disease; they may lack fever during an infection and pain in the case of a myocardial infarction. Instead, the elderly patient may present with general symptoms and signs such as delirium, falls, incontinence (with sudden start or rapid deterioration), or reduced intake of fluids leading to dehydration. It is most important that these symptoms are not interpreted as "normal aging"; aging does not happen overnight, and whenever there is an abrupt change in the functional or cognitive state of elderly patients, one must search systematically for an underlying cause.

Symptoms of cancer may be more difficult to interpret in the elderly because of comorbidity, and sometimes this leads to delayed diagnosis. Bone pain caused by a tumor may be interpreted as exacerbation of osteoarthritis, a brain tumor may be interpreted as dementia, and changes in bowel function are interpreted as constipation. In a patient with dementia who is not able to express pain or other problems distinctly, diagnosing cancer is even more difficult.

When cancer is diagnosed, treatment decisions will often be more complicated in the elderly patient because of several factors, such as reduced remaining life expectancy, the competing risks from comorbidities, reduced treatment tolerance, and potential drug interactions in the presence of polypharmacy. The impact of treatment on the patient's functional status as well as transportation and caregiver issues need to be addressed. In addition, the heterogeneity of this population complicates the creation of "one size fits all" evidence-based guidelines.

Delirium

Delirium is an acute (hours to days) decline in attention and cognition and is reported to occur in 20% to 80% of cancer patients. Delirium is an underdiagnosed condition associated with functional decline, increased morbidity and mortality, as well as increased health care costs. Two core features separate delirium from dementia.

- First, in delirium the cognitive failure develops rapidly, whereas in dementia it develops gradually.
- Second, delirium, but not dementia, is associated with impaired or fluctuating consciousness.
- Moreover, delirium is associated with an altered psychomotor activity.
  - ⌐ When the psychomotor activity is increased (hyperactive delirium), the patient is agitated, sometimes with hallucinations, with a marked motor hyperactivity, and may be difficult to manage.

┐ In the case of decreased psychomotor activity (hypoactive delirium), the patient is usually lying silently in his bed, but an attempt to communicate with him will reveal a severe confusion.

Most delirious patients fluctuate between hyperactive and hypoactive periods during the day. A general characteristic of delirium is its fluctuating course, making the condition difficult to diagnose.

The cause of delirium is multifactorial. If the patient is vulnerable because of cognitive impairment or several comorbidities, delirium could be triggered by a small event such as the introduction of a sleeping pill. Conversely, if the patient has few risk factors for delirium, the precipitating factors leading to delirium need to be more extreme such as surgery or major infections. Examples of risk factors for delirium are chronic cognitive dysfunction, high age, serious comorbidity, malnutrition, and sensory impairment.

Common precipitating factors are infections, dehydration, myocardial infarction, pulmonary embolism, urinary retention, renal failure, electrolyte disturbances, and the introduction of anticholinergic drugs. The introduction of opioid analgesics may also precipitate delirium, but pain and insufficient analgesia seem to be a more common precipitating factor.

During the search for the underlying cause of delirium, it is essential to keep in mind the atypical presentation of diseases in the elderly. A review of the patient's medications is mandatory. The most important therapeutic measure is to diagnose and treat the precipitating cause(s) if at all possible.

- Nonpharmacological interventions include the use of orienting influences such as a clock, regular reorienting communication, encouraging normal wake-sleep cycles, and involving family members in care.
- Pharmacological treatment may be necessary if the patient is a danger to himself or others, and haloperidol (orally or intravenously administered) is usually the agent of choice with doses of 0.5 to 1.0 mg twice daily with additional doses every four hours when necessary. An important side effect of haloperidol is extrapyramidal symptoms, and the use of this drug must be reduced to a minimum. Haloperidol is contraindicated in patients with dementia with Lewy bodies or Parkinson's disease.

In these patients, short-acting sedatives like oxazepam may constitute an alternative.

Dementia

According to the ICD-10 operational criteria, all the following must be fulfilled to make a diagnosis of dementia: there must be impairment in memory and at least one other cognitive function (e.g., language, visuospatial function, or logical reasoning). This impairment must be to a degree that interferes with the person's daily functioning. There must also be impairment of mental functions such as emotional control, motivation, or social behavior. The duration of the symptoms must be at least six months, and the consciousness must be normal.

The most common cause of dementia is Alzheimer disease, followed by vascular changes. Recent research has documented that the combination of Alzheimer and vascular pathology is more common than formerly believed. Other causes of dementia are Lewy body disease, with pronounced motor symptoms in addition to the cognitive failure and a marked intolerance for antipsychotic drugs, and frontotemporal dementia with dominating loss of emotional and behavioral control.

Most cases of dementia progress over several years from a mild impairment, which does not interfere with the person's ability to give an informed consent or to follow up cancer treatment, to severe stages making the person totally helpless in which palliative care should be prioritized.

Falls

An estimated one-third of persons over the age of 65 fall each year, and about half of the cases experience recurrent falls. Approximately 1 in 10 falls leads to a serious injury such as hip fracture or head injury. As seen in other geriatric syndromes, the risk of falls is multifactorial, and some of the most common risk factors include muscle weakness, history of falls, gait deficits, and balance deficits. Medications that may increase the fall risk include benzodiazepines, opioid analgesics, sleeping medication, and antidepressants.

Anticancer therapy often leads to an increased fall risk, examples being surgical treatment involving prolonged bed rest, which again leads to muscle loss and orthostatic hypotension, neurological side effects of chemotherapy, and pain treatment with opioid analgesics.

Two relevant clinical points are that patients often forget that they have fallen, and that they rarely volunteer the information about a fall even if they do remember it. It is thus important to ask the patient and caregiver about falls and to assess balance and gait when indicated.

Polypharmacy

Polypharmacy is most commonly defined as the regular use of five or more drugs but may also be defined as using medications that are not clinically indicated. Among home-dwelling persons over the age of 65, 39% use five or more drugs. Polypharmacy is not a bad thing per se. It has been documented that elderly patients are undertreated for many conditions, examples being atrial fibrillation and hypertension. On the other hand, a higher number of drugs increase the risk of interactions and adverse drug reactions.

A diagnosis of cancer will often necessitate a critical revision of the patient's drug list. For example, cancer may bring about changes in life expectancy that will deem some preventive drugs unnecessary, and the use of chemotoxic agents or other anticancer drugs increases the risk of drug-drug interactions.

Declaration of Interest:

Dr Kristjansson has reported no conflicts of interest.

Dr Wyller has reported that he has given lectures on different geriatric topics sponsored by Pfizer, Lundbeck and Roche.

Further Reading

Arking R. The Biology of Aging: Observations and Principles. 3rd ed. New York: Oxford University Press, 2006.

Finkel T, Serrano M, Blasco MA. The common biology of cancer and ageing. Nature 2007; 448:767–774.

Inouye SK. Delirium in older persons. N Engl J Med 2006; 354:1157–1165.

Tinetti ME. Clinical practice. Preventing falls in elderly persons. N Engl J Med 2003; 348:42–49.

Cancer Epidemiology

D. Schrijvers

*Department of Hemato-Oncology, Ziekenhuisnetwerk
Antwerpen-Middelheim, Antwerp, Belgium*

Introduction

Demography will change dramatically over the next 20 years and will influence the need for health care. An increasing proportion of people will be living longer, and there will be an increase in cancer prevalence. These changes will coincide with increasing dependency ratios and decreasing fertility rates in both developed and developing countries. This will influence the cancer care and treatment of the cancer patient who will be more isolated, frailer, and of an older age category.

Population Demographics

The proportion of the population aged 65 years or over will increase rapidly over the coming decades, augmented by the large cohort of "baby boomers" born in the two decades after the Second World War. There will be an increase in elderly people during the projected time period with a relative decrease in the number of people in the industrialized countries.

The life expectancy of people will also increase: according to the World Health Organisation (WHO), 26 countries will have a life expectancy at birth of above 80 years in the year 2025. It will be highest in Iceland, Italy, Japan, and Sweden (82 years) followed by Australia, Canada, France, Greece, The Netherlands, Singapore, Spain, and Switzerland (81 years). It will be 80 years in Austria, Belgium, Barbados, Costa Rica, Cyprus, Finland, Germany, Ireland, Israel, Luxembourg, Malta, New Zealand, the United Kingdom, and the United States. Other examples for 2025 include China (75 years), the Russian Federation (72 years), and India (71 years). The countries with the lowest life expectancies in 2025 will be Angola, Burkina Faso, Burundi, Chad, Mozambique, Niger, and Somalia (60 years); Mali and Uganda (59 years); Gambia and Guinea (58 years);

Table I Population Projections for the World and Different Regions

Year	Population in millions	
	2010	2050
World	6.909	9.150
Africa	1.033	1.998
Asia	4.167	5.231
Europe	733	691
Latin America and the Caribbean	589	729
Northern America	352	448
Oceania	36	51

Source: Population Division of the Department of Economic and Social Affairs of the United Nations Secretariat (2009). World population prospects: the 2008 revision. United Nations, New York.

Afghanistan, Malawi, and Rwanda (57 years); and Guinea Bissau (56 years) and Sierra Leone (51 years).

These reasons make that globally, the number of persons aged 60 or over is expected almost to triple, increasing from 737 million in 2009 to 2 billion by 2050. Furthermore, already 64% of the world's older persons live in less developed regions, and by 2050, 79% will do so.

Population projection in the different world regions and the proportion of people older than 60 and 80 years are given in Tables 1 and 2, respectively.

Cancer Demographics

Cancer is primarily a disease of old age. According to the National Cancer Institute (NCI), 60% of newly diagnosed malignancies are found in people over the age of 65 years. The same age group accounts for 70% of cancer deaths. Overall, the elderly are 10 times more likely to get cancer and 15 times more likely to die from cancer than people under the age of 65 years.

Table 2 *Proportion of the Population Aged over 65 and over 80*

	Age	2010	2050
World	Over 60	11	22
	Over 80	2	4
Africa	Over 60	5	11
	Over 80	0	1
Asia	Over 60	10	24
	Over 80	1	4
Europe	Over 60	22	34
	Over 80	4	10
Latin America and the Caribbean	Over 60	10	26
	Over 80	1	5
Northern America	Over 60	18	28
	Over 80	4	8
Oceania	Over 60	15	24
	Over 80	3	7

Source: Population Division of the Department of Economic and Social Affairs of the United Nations Secretariat (2009). World population prospects: the 2008 revision. United Nations, New York.

If all other factors remain the same, the demographic changes (population growth and an increasingly higher percentage of older individuals in the world population) will lead to a global increase of cancer incidence. By using the GLOBOCAN 2002 database, this results in 6,993,778 men diagnosed with cancer (increase of 20.5%) and 6,037,753 women (increase of 19.3%) in 2010.

Projections by the WHO state that because of the increase in cancer incidence, cancer mortality will increase to 12 million people by the year 2030 (Fig. 1).

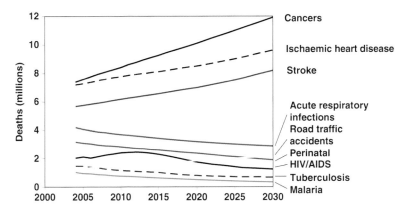

Figure 1   Global projections for selected causes from 2004 to 2030.

Since cancer treatment has become more effective, the number of cancer survivors and the prevalence of cancer in the population will also increase.

Society-Related Problems

Since there will be an increase in the number of cancer patients, the number of health care professionals to take care of these cancer patients will have to increase.

Projections by the NCI show that between 2005 and 2020 in the United States, there will be a 55.8% increase in the demand for oncologists, while in reality there will be a 14.5% increase in oncologists, leaving a gap of approximately 4,000 oncologists for the United States alone.

Other projections show that within the economically active population, there should be an increase of the health workers from 10% to 15% to maintain current levels of care.

The costs of cancer care and treatment will increase in the future, and this poses a heavy burden on the health care budgets of the different societies. The question remains if we will be able in the future to provide optimal cancer care and treatment within a reasonable cost-benefit model.

Conclusions

Because of the demographic changes and the fact that cancer is a disease of senior patients, more elderly cancer patients will need care and treatment. For an elderly cancer patient living with cancer, two issues are of special importance.

- Independence. Older people are interested in living long years, but they are even more interested in living independently and being able to do things. This means that efforts are needed within the society enabling older persons to remain independent as long as possible.
- Fragmentation of care. With older people, fragmentation of care can become a problem for treatment and care. Several different health care professionals will take care of these patients, and integration of a multidisciplinary approach between oncologists, geriatrician, and primary care physicians is of the utmost importance.

Declaration of Interest:

Dr Schrijvers has not reported any conflicts of interest.

Further Reading

Hayat MJ, Howlader N, Reichman ME, et al. Cancer statistics, trends, and multiple primary cancer analyses from the Surveillance, Epidemiology, and End Results (SEER) Program. Oncologist 2007; 12:20–37.

Matthews Z, Channon A. Will there be enough people to care? Notes on workforce implications of demographic change 2005–2050. World Health Organization, Geneva, 2006.

United Nations. World population prospects. The 2008 revision. United Nations, New York, 2009.

World Health Organisation. Boyle P, Levin B, eds. World Cancer Report. Lyon, France, 2008.

Evaluation of the Senior Cancer Patient: Comprehensive Geriatric Assessment and Screening Tools for the Elderly

M. Extermann
Moffitt Cancer Center, Tampa, Florida, U.S.A.

Introduction

Ageing being the main risk factor for cancer, most cancer patients are elderly. Several of these patients have accompanying comorbidities or geriatric problems (Table 1). In an oncology setting, not all of these problems might need a comprehensive approach beyond what would be done in the general adult population.

In our experience, half of patients aged 70 and older are functionally "old adults" and can be treated with a standard oncologic approach. The other half, however, will need more comprehensive care, including a comprehensive geriatric assessment (CGA).

The challenge for the oncologist is to distinguish between these two populations. Recent and ongoing research in geriatric oncology has started identifying effective short screening tools that are usable in a busy setting. Some of them were actually tested in emergency rooms and then adapted to oncology. The general workup of an older cancer patient is outlined in Figure 1.

One should note the importance of doing an early geriatric screening. This allows using the two to four weeks usually needed for an oncology workup for a parallel geriatric workup if necessary, with the impact on treatment outlined in Figure 2. In this chapter a few examples of screening tools for which effectiveness data specific to older cancer patients are available are

Table 1 *Prevalence of Problems in Older Cancer Patients: Outpatient Oncology Clinic Setting*

Problems	Prevalence (%)
ECOG PS $\geq$ 2	~20
ADL dependence	~20
IADL dependence	50–60
Comorbidity	>90
Severe comorbidity	30–40
Depression	20–40
Cognitive impairment	25–35
At risk of malnutrition/malnourished	30–50

Abbreviations: ECOG, Eastern Cooperative Oncology Group; PS, performance score; ADL, activities of daily living; IADL, instrumental activities of daily living.

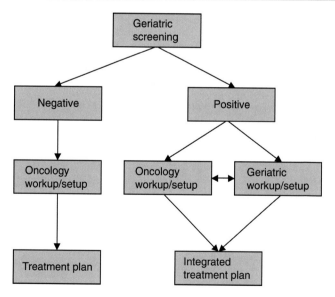

Figure 1 *General approach to treatment planning in an older cancer patient.*

Assessment tree and treatment strategy for elderly patients

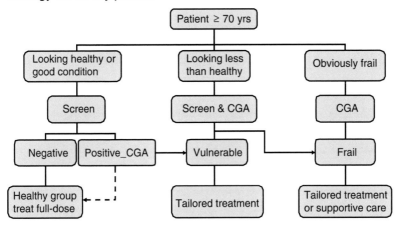

CGA, comprehensive geriatric assessment

Figure 2   Treatment approach based on levels of geriatric impairment.

discussed. They can be divided into two groups: short screening tools and multidimensional geriatric assessment (MGA) packages.

Short Screening Tools

These are rapid triage tools taking only a few minutes to answer. Their performance is compared in Table 2.

The Abbreviated CGA

Overcash et al. isolated 15 items (an abbreviated CGA) that correlated with the findings of an MGA in a large database of older patients with cancer who underwent a CGA as part of their oncology evaluation. These 15 items include three questions about activities of daily living (ADL), four questions about instrumental activities of daily living (IADL), four questions from the Mini-Mental Status (MMS) Examination, and four questions from the Geriatric Depression Scale (GDS).

Table 2 *Comparative Performance of CGA Screening Tools Vs. a Comprehensive Evaluation in Cancer Patients*

Tool	Sensitivity	Specificity	PPV	NPV
aCGA[a]	0.84–0.96	0.81–0.821	–	–
SAOP2				
Complete	100%	40%	90%	100%
W/o comorbidity	91%	44%	80%	67%
TRST	92.9%	–	67.7%	87.5%
VES 13	72.7%	85.7%	88.9%	66.7%

[a]Overall correlation with full scales: 0.84–0.96.
Abbreviations: PPV, positive predictive value; NPV, negative predictive value; CGA, comprehensive geriatric assessment; aCGA, abbreviated comprehensive geriatric assessment; SAOP2, Senior Adult Oncology Program 2 screening tool; W/o, with or without; TRST, Triage Risk Screening Tool; VES 13, Vulnerable Elders Survey 13.

If the patient has any impairment in the ADL or IADL items in the abbreviated CGA, then the full ADL and IADL scales should be administered. If two depression items are altered, a full GDS should be administered. A score of 6 or less in the cognitive screen triggers a full MMS. The score can be obtained from the article by Overcash in 2005.

The Senior Adult Oncology Program 2 Screening Tool

The Senior Adult Oncology Program (SAOP) 2 screening tool (Fig. 3) is an empirical tool that was developed by the multidisciplinary clinical team of the SAOP at Moffitt to determine when a multidisciplinary team consultation was required in new patients. In addition to function, depression, and cognitive screening, the screen includes questions regarding quality of life, self-rated health, falls, nutrition, sleep, polymedication, and social questions (drug payment and caregiver availability).

After more than five years of clinical use, this screen has demonstrated face validity, finding that 63% of senior cancer patients needed psychosocial counseling, 40% dietary intervention, and 14% medication counseling and assistance (the latter probably underestimated).

Name:_____ UR#_____ Age:_____

Diagnosis:_____ MD_____

1. If it was necessary, is there someone who could help take   Yes   No
   care of you?
2. Do you feel sad more days than not?   Yes   No
3. Have you lost interest in things you used to enjoy (hobbies,   Yes   No
   food, sex, being with friends/family)?
4. On a scale of 1 to 10, rate your present quality of life (10 is the best life, 1 is the
   worst)

     1   2   3   4   5   6   7   8   9   10
   worst   best

5. On a scale of 1 to 10, rate your present overall health (10 is the excellent, 1 is
   the poor)

1   2   3   4   5   6   7   8   9   10
[Poor   ]   [Fair   ]   [Good]   [Excellent]

6. Activities of Daily Living:

Can you dress yourself completely?........	Yes	Yes but with help	No
Can you feed yourself?	Yes	Yes but with help	No
Do you use a cane, walker, or wheelchair?.	Yes	Yes occasionally	No
Do you need help to get out of bed/chair?.	Yes	Yes but with help	No
Are you incontinent of urine?...............	Yes	Occasionally	No
Do you need help taking a shower or a bath?	Yes	Occasionally	No
Have you tripped or fallen in the past year?	Yes		No
Are you able to drive?.........................	Yes	Have Never Driven	No
Are you able to prepare your own meals?.	Yes	Yes but with help	No
Are you able to go shopping?	Yes	Yes but with help	No
Can you take care of your finances?	Yes	Yes but with help	No
Can you use the telephone?	Yes	Yes but with help	No
Do you remember to take your medications?......................................	Yes	Yes but with help	No

7. Have you lost 5 or more pounds in the past 6 months without   Yes   No
   dieting?
8. Has your appetite decreased in the last 3 months?   Yes   No

Figure 3   Senior Adult Oncology Program 2 screening questionnaire.

9. Has there been a change in the <u>types</u> of foods you are able to eat? Yes No

10. Are you always able to pay for your prescription medications? Yes No

11. Do you feel you are sleeping well? Yes No

Please stop here. Thank you!

***I am going to name 3 objects (pencil, truck, book) and ask you to repeat them now and a few minutes from now to test your memory.

12. Spell the word "clown" backwards. n-w-o-l-c .... 5 points = _____

13. What is today's date and day? Mth.___Date___Yr.___, Day____ .... 4 points = _____

14. Can you repeat the 3 objects I mentioned earlier? I[ ] 2[ ] 3[ ] .... 3 points = _____

                                                                        Total = _____

15. How many medications/herbals/vitamins are you taking? _____ .... None [ ]

Additional information:

ECOG PS:_____   Usual weight=_____   Current weight=_____

Nutrition: BMI_____   MNAs_____   Referral: No Yes

SW: GDS_____   MMSE_____   Referral: No Yes

Figure 3 Continued

Its performance was validated against an MGA (Table 2). The first page is answered directly by the patient, and the second page is administered by the clinic staff. If one item is positive, the respective specialist is called in. If several items are impaired, the multidisciplinary team is called in or a geriatric referral is made for a CGA.

The Triage Risk Screening Tool

The Triage Risk Screening Tool (TRST) (Fig. 4) was developed for geriatric screening in the emergency room setting. Patients screening positive then underwent a half-hour evaluation by a geriatric nurse practitioner.

Cognitive decline	2
Lives alone or no caregiver	1
Restricted mobility or fall within last six months	1
Hospitalization within last three months	1
Polypharmacy (≥5 drugs)	1
Any positive item would warrant geriatric evaluation in cancer patients.	

Figure 4 The Triage Risk Screening Tool.

Its performance was compared with a full CGA in oncology patients (Kenis et al.). It proved sensitive provided the threshold was lowered from 2 to 1 point. Therefore, any positive item would warrant geriatric evaluation in cancer patients.

The Vulnerable Elders Survey 13

Mohile et al. analyzed the performance of the Vulnerable Elders Survey (VES) 13, developed in a large geriatric survey cohort, in older prostate cancer patients. Fifty percent of patients were identified as impaired on the VES 13 (score ≥ 3). That cutoff had a sensitivity of 72.7% and a specificity of 85.7% for impairment in two or more dimensions on an MGA (Table 2). The score can be obtained from, for example, http://www.usafp.org/Word_PDF_Files/Best-Practices/Vulnerable%20Elders%20Survey.doc.

MGA Packages

MGA packages are sets of a half dozen questionnaires or tests aimed at providing an overall geriatric evaluation in the study setting, a second step in patients screening positive on short screens, a preoperative evaluation, or a first evaluation in an obviously frail patient. They usually screen for functional and cognitive impairments, depression, malnutrition, and comorbidity, using validated geriatric instruments. A couple of study-specific questionnaires can easily be added for an overall evaluation time of about 20 minutes. Some examples are as follows:

▪ Katz ADL, Lawton's nine-item IADL, Eastern Cooperative Oncology Group (ECOG) performance status (PS), GDS (15 items), Folstein's

MMS, Mini-Nutritional Assessment (MNA), Cumulative Illness Rating Scale—Geriatric (CIRS-G). Used, for example, in Moffitt and Radiation Therapy Oncology Group (RTOG) studies.

- ADL (MOS physical health), IADL (Older Americans' Resources and Services subscale), timed getup and go, comorbidity (OARS subscale), Blessed Orientation Memory-Concentration Test, Hospital Anxiety-Depression Scale (HADS), MOS social functioning and support subscales, body mass index (BMI), and weight loss. Used, for example, in Cancer and Leukemia Group B (CALGB) studies.
- Katz ADL, Lawton's IADL, ECOG PS, MMS, GDS, comorbidity (CIRS-G or Satariano), and EORTC-QLQ30/social support. Used, for example, in European Organization for Research and Treatment of Cancer (EORTC) or Gruppo Italiano di Oncologia Geriatrica (GIOGer) studies.
- Katz ADL, Lawton's IADL, ECOG PS, GDS, MMS, Brief Fatigue Inventory, comorbidity (Satariano), American Society of Anesthesiologists (ASA) score. Used, for example, by the International Society of Geriatric Oncology (SIOG) Surgical Task Force.

The component instruments are available in several languages through online sources.

Declaration of Interest:

Prof Extermann has reported no conflicts of interest.

Further Reading

Extermann M, Green T, Tiffenberg G, et al. Validation of the Senior Adult Oncology Program (SAOP) 2 screening questionnaire. Crit Rev Oncol Hematol 2009; 69:185.

Extermann M, Hurria A. Comprehensive geriatric assessment for older patients with cancer. J Clin Oncol 2007; 25:1824–1831.

Johnson D, Blair J, Balducci L, et al. The assessment of clinical resources in a senior adult oncology program. European Oncology Nursing Society Meeting, Innsbruck, Austria, 2006.

Kenis C, Geeraerts A, Braesl T, et al. The Flemish version of the Triage Risk Screening Tool (TRST): a multidimensional short screening tool for the assessment of elderly patients. Crit Rev Oncol Hematol 2006; 60:S31.

Mion LC, Palmer RM, Anetzberger GJ, et al. Establishing a case-finding and referral system for at-risk older individuals in the emergency department setting: the SIGNET model. J Am Geriatr Soc 2001; 49:1379–1386.

Mohile SG, Bylow K, Dale W, et al. A pilot study of the vulnerable elders survey-13 compared with the comprehensive geriatric assessment for identifying disability in older patients with prostate cancer who receive androgen ablation. Cancer 2007; 109:802–810.

Overcash JA, Beckstead J, Extermann M, et al. The abbreviated comprehensive geriatric assessment (aCGA): a retrospective analysis. Crit Rev Oncol Hematol 2005; 54:129–136.

Overcash JA, Beckstead J, Moody L, et al. The abbreviated comprehensive geriatric assessment (aCGA) for use in the older cancer patient as a prescreen: scoring and interpretation. Crit Rev Oncol Hematol 2006; 59:205–210.

Saliba D, Orlando M, Wenger NS, et al. Identifying a short functional disability screen for older persons. J Gerontol A Biol Sci Med Sci 2000; 55:M750–M756.

Frailty in the Elderly

M. Gosney

University of Reading, Reading, Berkshire, U.K.

Frailty in the Elderly

Frailty is a physiological syndrome, which is characterized clinically by decreased reserve and diminished resistance to stressors, which has resulted from cumulative decline across multiple physiological systems during ageing. It places older people at risk for death and other adverse health outcomes. Many of the outcomes that are associated with frailty are fractures, hospitalization, and a new onset or a worsening of a previous diminished capacity to perform various activities of daily living. Fried and coworkers, in 2001, used data from over 5,000 men and women aged 65 years or older, who had been recruited between 1989 and 1990 into a cardiovascular health study, to suggest that although frailty had previously been considered to be synonymous with disability, comorbidity, and other clinical characteristics, it must also be recognized to have a biologic basis and to be a distinct clinical syndrome. They characterized the clinical syndrome of frailty when three or more of the following criteria were present: greater than 10 lb or 4.5 kg unintentional weight loss in the previous year, self-reported exhaustion, slow walking speed, low physical activity, and weakness, as measured by grip strength. A prevalence of approximately 7% was found in their community-dwelling population, which increased with age and was also more common in women than in men.

In 2008 Ravaglia and colleagues developed a prognostic score for frailty outcomes in older people. In their study of over 1,000 Italian subjects, they evaluated 17 baseline possible mortality predictors and compared these with four-year risk mortality and adverse health outcomes usually associated with frailty. Table 1 shows the nine predictors of mortality.

Although some of the factors listed in Table 1 were not independent predictors of mortality, the multivariate adjusted model included only the

Table 1 *Univariate Analysis of Potential Predictors for Four-Year Mortality*

Variable (number of subjects)	Number of deaths (%)	HR (95% CI)	P value
Demographic age (years)			
<80 (761)	60 (7.9)	1	–
≥80 (246)	87 (35.4)	4.99 (3.59–6.95)	<0.001
Gender			
Women (558)	78 (14.0)	1	–
Men (449)	69 (15.4)	1.15 (0.83–1.59)	0.391
Physical inactivity			
No (554)	31 (5.6)	1	–
Yes (453)	116 (25.6)	5.00 (3.36–7.42)	<0.001
Daily use of ≥3 drugs			
No (635)	64 (10.1)	1	–
Yes (372)	83 (22.3)	2.37 (1.71–3.29)	<0.001
Sensory deficits			
No (970)	131 (13.5)	1	–
Yes (37)	16 (43.2)	4.13 (2.46–6.94)	<0.001
Nutritional status			
Calf circumference, cm			
≥31 (821)	90 (11.0)	1	–
<31 (186)	57 (30.6)	3.05 (2.18–4.26)	<0.001
Functional status			
Instrumental activities of daily living			
No difficulty (810)	69 (8.5)	1	–
Any difficulty (197)	78 (39.6)	5.25 (3.79–7.27)	<0.001
Gait and balance test score			
>24 (759)	58 (7.6)	1	–
≤24 (248)	89 (35.9)	5.24 (3.77–7.30)	0.001

(Continued)

Table 1 *Univariate Analysis of Potential Predictors for Four-Year Mortality (Continued)*

Variable (number of subjects)	Number of deaths (%)	HR (95% CI)	P value
Pessimism about one's own health	–	–	–
No (863)	99 (11.5)	1	–
Yes (144)	48 (33.3)	3.25 (2.30–4.59)	<0.001

Abbreviations: HR, hazard ration; CI, confidence interval.
Source: Adapted from Ravaglia et al., 2008.

Table 2 *Four-Year Risk of Mortality According to Individual Prognostic Scores*

Prognostic score	Number of subjects	Number of deaths	(% of groups)
0–2	628	32	5.1
3	159	19	11.9
4	83	18	21.7
5	61	25	41.0
6	49	32	65.3
≥7	27	21	77.8

Source: Adapted from Ravaglia et al., 2008.

nine predictors listed in Table 1. The presence of increasing numbers of these nine items showed an increased risk factor. Those scoring 0 had a 5.1% four-year mortality versus a 77.8% four-year mortality in those who scored 7 or greater (Table 2).

A score of 4 or greater on this prognostic scoring system was associated with four-year risks of fracture (12%), hospital admission (28%), worsening disability (60%), and incident disability (63%).

While frailty has five clearly defined components, unintentional weight loss, self-reported fatigue, diminished physical activity, and measured impairment, (when compared with age-standardized norms of both grip strength and gait speed), it fails to consider cognitive and psychosocial features, which are not only predictive of adverse health outcomes but may also be particularly prevalent in older people with cancer.

There have been a number of suggestions for "different culprits" that cause frailty. Cytokines and other components of the inflammatory response are possibly implicated, but this has not always been consistent. Hubbard and colleagues have found that the frailty index correlates significantly with a log-transformed C-reactive protein and interleukin (IL)-6 and with absolute values of tumor necrosis factor α (TNF-α) and correlated inversely with measured serum albumin.

Many older people with cancer will have coexisting frailty; however, very few studies look at the true prevalence of defined frailty rather than the presence of a "frail" individual. Mohile, using data from the 2003 Medicate Current Beneficiary Survey, studied almost 12,500 community dwelling elders in the United States. The aim of the study was to evaluate whether cancer was independently associated with vulnerability and frailty. They used criteria as defined by Balducci for frailty and the Vulnerable Elders Survey 13 (VES 13) but did not use the measures of frailty as defined by Fried and widely used by geriatricians. When compared with an age-matched control group, those with a history of cancer were more likely to have limitations of activities of daily living, higher prevalence of geriatric syndromes, lower self-related health, higher scores on the VES 13, and a more frequent diagnosis of "frailty" (Table 3).

The Impact of Frailty on Cancer

There is little doubt that frailty affects the cancer patient at three specific time periods.

▪ Initially, when the patient presents, the coexistence of frailty with a new diagnosis of cancer may result in uncertainty as to how aggressive the planned therapy should be. Patients with underlying correctable frailty, for example, nutritional deficiencies that have occurred as a result of cancer, may be undertreated or even denied treatment if the clinician is not aware of the reversibility of the condition causing the frailty. However, in contrast, patients who have frailty due to advanced

Table 3 *Cancer Diagnosis Association After Adjustment for Confounders*

Low self-rated health	
OR	1.46
CI 95	1.30–1.64
RR	1.33
Limitations in activities of daily living	
OR	1.19
CI 95%	1.06–1.33
RR	1.13
Limitations in instrumental activities of daily living	
OR	1.25
CI 95%	1.13–1.38
RR	1.13
Geriatric syndrome	
OR	1.27
CI 95%	1.15–1.41
RR	1.11
VES 13 score of 3 or higher	
OR	1.26
CI 95%	1.13–1.41
RR	1.14
Frailty (Balducci criteria)	
OR	1.46
CI 95%	1.29–1.65
RR	1.09

Abbreviations: OR, adjusted odds ratio; CI, confidence interval; RR, relative risk; VES 13, Vulnerable Elders Survey 13.
Source: Adapted from Mohile et al., 2009.

coexisting diseases may be more suited for palliative rather than curative cancer therapy, and conditions such as end-stage cardio-respiratory disease prior to the detection of cancer may result in death "with" rather than "from" cancer.

- Secondly, during therapy for cancer, coexisting frailty may increase the risk of therapy associated toxicity, may reduce quality of life and therefore discourage the older patient from continuing with therapy, or may result in either cancer- or non-cancer-related "geriatric" syndromes.

- Finally, during the follow-up period post cancer treatment, the development of or worsening of existing frailty may reduce overall survival, although it should not affect disease-free survival.

Assessment of Frailty

Until recently, both geriatricians and oncologists developed assessment methodologies predominantly designed for their individual patient populations. A review of a clinical assessment of elderly people with cancer in 2005 highlighted many of the deficiencies of the different assessment methodologies. With more recent collaborative work between the two groups, the role of comprehensive geriatric assessment (CGA) is now being well validated. The CGA has become increasingly accepted, and by using such assessment methodologies, Retornaz has validated the use of seven frailty markers (nutrition, mobility, strength, energy, physical activity, mood, and cognition) and found that nutrition, mobility, and physical activity were the most prevalent in a group of older individuals referred for chemotherapy. In addition, up to 42% of older cancer patients had areas of potential vulnerability that would not have been detected through the more traditionally used instrumental activity of daily living (IADL) and activity of daily living (ADL). While mobility and physical activity are well-known predictors of morbidity and mortality in frailty studies, the addition of nutrition is important, particularly in a cancer patient. It is gratifying to see both mood and cognition included since the latter is one of the "giants of geriatric medicine," as described initially by Bernard Issacs. There is, however, little in the cancer literature about the role of sensory deprivation due to impaired vision and hearing, acute delirium, both fecal and urinary incontinence, and impaired gait and falls on the management of cancer.

Conclusion

There is little doubt that frailty exists and that its diagnosis is fraught with problems in the cancer patient. Oncologists and geriatricians use different definitions of frailty, may measure functional status with different assessment tools, and may see very different patients. Frailty may be reversible in some patients, and the oncologist needs to work toward identifying the presence of such factors as nutritional deficiency, poor mobility, incontinence, and delirium both before and during therapy. Patients suitable for therapy require comprehensive assessment with validated tools, and the word "frail" should not exclude individuals from potentially life-saving therapy. Follow-up should include an active search for remediable problems that are often not cancer related. Finally, when recording the cause of death in older patients, cancer should not be cited as a cause of death unless clear evidence of its presence and contribution to a patient's decline exists.

Declaration of Interest:

Prof Gosney has reported no conflicts of interest.

Further Reading

Fried LP, Tangen CM, Walston J, et al. Frailty in older adults: evidence for a phenotype. Gerontol A Biol Sci Med Sci 2001; 56(3):M146–M156.

Gosney MA. Clinical assessment of elderly people with cancer. Lancet Oncol 2005; 6:790–797.

Hubbard RE, O'Mahony MS, Savva GM, et al. Inflammation and frailty measures in older people. J Cell Mol Med 2009; [Epub ahead of print].

Mohile SG, Xian Y, Dale W, et al. Association of a cancer diagnosis with vulnerability and frailty in older Medicare beneficiaries. J Natl Cancer Inst 2009; 101(17):1206–1215.

Ravaglia G, Forti P, Lucicesare A, et al. Development of an easy prognostic score for frailty outcomes in the aged. Age Ageing 2008; 37:161–166.

Retornaz F, Monette J, Batist G, et al. Usefulness of frailty markers in the assessment of the health and functional status of older cancer patients referred for chemotherapy: a pilot study. J Gerontol A Biol Sci Med Sci 2008; 63(5): 518–522.

Surgical Treatment

5

S. Gaskell
Mersey Deanery, Liverpool, Merseyside, U.K.

R.A. Audisio
Department of Surgery, University of Liverpool, St Helens & Knowsley Teaching Hospitals, St Helens, Merseyside, U.K.

Introduction

Surgical removal currently represents the treatment of choice for most solid tumors regardless of the patients' age. A robust body of evidence supports this, and it was clearly demonstrated that long-term cancer-related survival is comparable between different age cohorts. An accurate comparison of different series demonstrated no inferiority in survival in the older age group, although the presence of a selection bias that favours geriatric series should be considered.

Indications for Surgery

Beyond curative excisions, surgical oncologists play a major role in the palliation of cancer patients. As for younger patients, a palliative procedure is indicated when: (*i*) general health status is acceptable, (*ii*) the condition is likely to be quickly reversible, and (*iii*) the patient is asking for surgical treatment and accepts the high operative risk. Alternatively, every effort should be put in place to improve quality of life and palliate symptoms with pharmaceutical intervention rather than with the use of tubes, drains, or catheters.

It is important to ensure that older cancer patients receive operations under elective conditions because operative morbidity and mortality dramatically increase with patient age in the emergency situation. Regrettably, the proportion of older cancer patients admitted as a surgical emergency requiring an urgent operation is higher than that in the younger group.

- For older gastric and colorectal cancer patients presenting with obstructive colorectal symptoms, the surgical death rate is three times higher than that of younger patients. Typically, this older cohort is most frequently treated with a diverting stoma, however, only 40% to 60% of such patients will have their stoma reversed. Self-expanding metallic stents are worth considering both for palliation and as a bridge to surgery in acute decompression of colonic obstruction where a less invasive alternative to a defunctioning colostomy or cecostomy allows appropriate resuscitation, correction of malnutrition, anemia, and hydroelectrolytic rebalancing. A recent cost analysis comparison of stents versus surgery has shown that colonic stents result in 23% fewer operative procedures per patient (1.01 vs. 1.32 surgical procedures/patient), 83% reduction in stoma requirement (7% vs. 43%), and lower procedure-related mortality (5% vs. 11%).

A close collaboration with orthopedic surgeons has led to a novel approach in the management of cancer patients with bone metastases. Bone lesions are frequently considered for fixation and consolidation; these procedures can now be performed as day cases, and the patients' prompt recovery allows for early start of chemotherapy.

More and more cosmetic surgery is being performed on older patients to optimize body image after mutilating cancer surgery; this is not surprising since aesthetical outcomes are very important to older patients who are fit for cosmetic surgery and are seeking to regain full domain of their social functions. This is now often the case in breast reconstruction because of an increasing proportion of breast cancer in elderly patients accompanied by a decline in cancer mortality. Within any practice encompassing either immediate or delayed reconstruction, older patients potentially form a significant part of the eligible patient group. Despite many studies demonstrating fewer older women receiving breast reconstruction than younger ones (7–8.5% vs. 40–50%), it is likely that this proportion will be soon modified.

Patients Selection

A large body of clinical evidence has been collected, which demonstrates an unacceptable variation in the surgical management of older cancer patients. This variation is also reflected between more or less aggressive procedures, that is, older patients are more often undertreated or even not treated at all.

Older cancer patients represent a very diverse population, and it is crucial to frame each individual according to frailty to tailor treatment plans. This information is also mandatory when consenting older cancer patients and discussing the real advantages of a procedure against the risks it entails. Furthermore, there are a number of older individuals with cancer in whom a careful assessment may detect early-stage disability and geriatric syndromes, which could be treated promptly and reflect in better short-term outcomes.

Over the last decade, lessons have been learned from geriatricians, and the use of validated assessment tools is being considered in oncologic practice.

- It has been shown that a comprehensive geriatric assessment (CGA) adds substantial information on the functional assessment of older cancer patients, particularly those with a good performance scale (PS).
- The role of PS as the sole reliable marker of functional status has lost consistency for older cancer patients.
- The American Society of Anesthesiologists (ASA) score is helpful in predicting mortality on the general population but was not found to be predictive of postoperative complications and hospital stay.
- The Physiological and Operative Severity Score for Enumeration of Mortality and Morbidity (POSSUM) and its modification P-POSSUM have been prospectively validated, with the P-POSSUM formula designed to better predict operative mortality in cases where POSSUM overstated the observed mortality. POSSUM and P-POSSUM were also developed to predict outcomes; regrettably, the reliability is poor in the elderly subgroup, and most importantly, some information can only be retrieved peroperatively rather than before the decision is made to undergo surgery or consider medical palliation.
- It is only recently that CGA has been applied to an oncogeriatric surgical series in which 460 cases were prospectively entered into an observational study with the aim of defining the general health condition of senior cancer individuals (preoperative assessment of cancer in the elderly). Thirty-day morbidity is principally related to instrumental activities of daily living (IADL) and brief fatigue inventory (BFI), whereas the postoperative hospital stay correlates with activities of daily living (ADL).

- Computerized models for the prediction of postoperative mortality in older patients (>80 years) undergoing cancer surgery have been developed. Multivariate analysis identifying age, operative urgency, ASA grade, no cancer excision versus resection, and metastatic spread as independent risk factors have provided an initial model for specific colorectal procedures, in which there is a good correlation between observed and predicted outcomes.

At present, all efforts are being made to develop a reliable tool on the basis of previous experience, with the requisite of being quick and user friendly. The decision-making process would certainly benefit if patients were screened for frailty in clinic, with the more vulnerable ones requiring multidisciplinary management with geriatricians and specialist care. The ongoing PREOP research project is looking at the reliability of new assessment instruments, that is, Groningen Frailty Index, Vulnerable Elders Survey, or a functional assessment as the timed "up and go."

Outcomes

Bernard Isaacs described incontinence, instability and falls, impaired hearing and vision, and intellectual decline as the giants of geriatric medicine.

Comorbidities are highly relevant to the prognosis of cancer patients. They not only affect prognosis but also influence the treatment offered to the patients. This is in part due to the effect that additional comorbidities affect not only prognosis but also their influence on the treatment of such patients. Before embarking in any treatment planning with older patients, it is crucial to appreciate the patient's requests and expectations as these might be substantially different from what the care team was predicting.

Short-term outcomes are postoperative mortality, complications rate, and length of hospital stay. Technical skills, both surgical and anesthetic, may influence short-term outcomes. The operating team should be up to date with recent technical advancements and careful handling, but most importantly, older surgical cancer patients should be considered for early discharge (from hospital as well as intensive care units), prompt mobilization, early oral feeding, and the use of suprapubic urinary catheters in males, which has been shown to reduce urinary complications.

It is also important to realize how quality of life gains are an absolute priority in older subgroups. It is not possible to care for a stoma when one is shortsighted and suffering from arthritis. Sphincter-saving procedures as well as all alternative options such as transanal microscopic microsurgery should be considered. The same applies for any other operation that might cause significant disabilities.

Delirium is frequently reported as being highly prevalent in elderly surgical series, although most surgical teams are unaware of it because the time spent with the patient is so short that cognitive changes go undetected. The detection of delirium is important as its occurrence impacts on the length of hospital stay, morbidity, and mortality rates.

Survival

It is crucial to understand that state-of-the-art surgery is equally effective in older cancer patients as well younger ones when cancer-related survival is considered. On the other hand, as the elderly population has a shorter life expectancy, it comes with no surprise that large amounts of data confirm that the overall survival is reduced regardless of cancer site.

There is no reason not to offer standard surgical management to older patients provided the patient is not frail. Similarly, there is no need to diminish any standard of care unless proven otherwise. Rutten et al. analyzed population-based registries and suggested a negative impact of the recently introduced total mesorectal excision for rectal cancer in the older-age subgroup. It was suggested that frail senior individuals do not benefit from this extended procedure since it carries a high operative morbidity and mortality rate.

More clinical research is needed to tailor treatment to oncogeriatric series. Until this has occurred, it is not appropriate to offer substandard surgery or not to consider a definitive surgical operation.

Palliation

The surgical management of patients presenting with incurable cancers is controversial. Surgical treatment is often offered to optimize quality of life and prolong survival regardless of the patient's age. The controversy is further increased when the patient is elderly and his/her survival will inevitably be shorter than average. It is advisable to discuss targets with these patients and to clearly understand what their expectations are. Day-to-day wellbeing should, in any case, be prioritized and discussed with older patients, where the vast majority would like to be told of their diagnosis and prognosis. It has been shown how they generally seek an active involvement in the decision-making process regarding cancer therapy and most frequently opt for advanced management (i.e., breast-sparing surgery with adjuvant treatment when given the choice). As previously mentioned, the use of self-expandable metal stents represents an interesting strategy, particularly for patients presenting with a colonic stricture in an emergency setting. Aggressive surgical treatment of advanced obstructive disease has been advocated, but stenting is to be preferred until convincing data on improved quality of life is available.

Side Effects

When dealing with older individuals, it is important to appreciate how (*i*) minor complications (i.e., wound infection, leaks, seromas) may result in excessive discomfort related to the practical problems such as attending dressing clinics, transportation, and polypharmacy; and (*ii*) major complications (i.e., severe chest infection, sepsis, renal/liver failure) are more likely to result in a life-threatening condition because of a lower physiological threshold and poor immunological/nutritional status.

- Several minor complications are preventable: preoperative evidence of depression can be pharmacologically corrected to decrease postoperative delirium. Early discharge may reduce the incidence of methicillin-resistant *Staphylococcus aureus* (MRSA) infection, and the use of suprapubic urinary catheters successfully decreases the rate of urinary complications.
- Seroma/hematoma formation can be prevented by minimizing the flap preparation, by accurate dissection, and by meticulous hemostasis.
- Chest infection is the morbidity frequently associated with postoperative death; therefore, appropriate post-operative physiotherapy should always be implemented.

Conclusion

A modern oncogeriatric surgical service should be based on the assumption that senior cancer patients represent a different population in terms of physiological response, polypharmacy, psychological attitudes, and life expectations. The implementation of guidelines may be effective in reducing complications and mortality, but the use of tailored treatment planning is mandatory for this frail and rapidly expanding patient group.

Declaration of Interest:

Prof Audisio has reported no conflicts of interest.

Dr Gaskell has reported no conflicts of interest.

Further Reading

Audisio RA, Veronesi P, Ferrario L, et al. Elective surgery for gastrointestinal tumours in the elderly. Ann Oncol 1997; 8(4):317–326.

Heriot AG, Tekkis PP, Smith JJ, et al. Prediction of postoperative mortality in elderly patients with colorectal cancer. Dis Colon Rectum 2006; 49:816–824.

Morris E, Quirke P, Thomas JD, et al. Unacceptable variation in abdominoperineal excision rates for rectal cancer: time to intervene? Gut 2008; 57:1690–1697.

PACE participants. Shall we operate? Preoperative assessment in elderly cancer patients (PACE) can help—a SIOG surgical task force prospective study. Crit Rev Oncol Hematol 2008; 65:156–163.

Pope D, Ramesh H, Gennari R, et al. Pre-operative assessment of cancer in the elderly (PACE): a comprehensive assessment of underlying characteristics of elderly cancer patients prior to elective surgery. Surg Oncol 2006; 15:189–197.

Read WL, Tierney RM, Page NC, et al. Differential prognostic impact of comorbidity. J Clin Oncol 2004; 22:3099–3103.

Rutten HJ, den Dulk M, Lemmens VE, et al. Controversies of total mesorectal excision for rectal cancer in elderly patients. Lancet Oncol 2008; 9:494–501.

Targownik LE, Spiegel BM, Sack J, et al. Colonic stent vs. emergency surgery for management of acute left-sided malignant colonic obstruction: a decision analysis. Gastrointest Endosc 2004; 60:865–874.

Radiotherapy in the Elderly Cancer Patient

6

D.C. Christoph and W.E.E. Eberhardt

Department of Medicine (Cancer Research), West German Cancer Centre, University Hospital of the University Duisburg-Essen, Essen, Germany

Indications for Radiotherapy in the Elderly

Compared with other treatment modalities like surgery and combination chemotherapy, radiotherapy has the advantage of less severe side effects, especially rare treatment-related mortality. This becomes of particular importance in elderly or frail patients who typically present with a considerable number of clinically relevant comorbidities such as vascular problems (e.g., cardiovascular, cerebrovascular, or general arteriosclerotic vascular disease) or organ impairments [e.g., emphysema, chronic obstructive lung disease (COLD), renal insufficiency, and diabetes mellitus]. Radiotherapy represents a local modality that—in solid tumors—can be aimed at primary tumor (local disease) and involved regional lymph nodes (locoregional disease) as well as systemic points/regions of need (systemic metastases).

- In locally confined disease (early stages I/II), excellent results are achieved with aggressive higher radiation doses in curative intent (>60–70 Gray (Gy)). Considerable local control can be observed after even higher and more focused doses [stereotactic radiotherapy (SRT)].
- Locally advanced stages (e.g., III) in solid tumors are characterized by locoregional node involvement (N factor) or locoregional disease extension (T factor). Radiotherapy targets both primary, where usually higher doses are needed because of bulky disease areas, as well as locoregional lymph node areas, where reduced doses can still eradicate nodal disease. Thus, some patients can be cured with this locoregional treatment strategy. With cisplatin-based chemotherapy given concurrently with radiotherapy, even higher local efficacy/control can be induced.

- In metastasized, advanced stages, radiation doses of 30 to 50 Gy can still achieve excellent management for areas of need (e.g., brain, bone, soft tissue metastases). Reduction of clinical symptoms is the main palliative end point of these interventions.

While this simplified classification system describes a number of solid tumors (e.g., lung, rectal, prostate, breast cancer), hematological malignancies such as Hodgkin's disease, non-Hodgkin's lymphoma (NHL), and plasmocytoma have more specific treatment protocols where systemic modalities have gained increasingly important roles in curative management (e.g., innovative chemoimmunotherapy in NHL), while radiation has decreased in its indications based on toxicity issues in some (Hodgkin's disease) but still remains a valuable palliative and symptomatic care for others.

When prognostic factors such as performance status (PS) or pretreatment weight loss are taken into account, older patients are usually treated with more intensive protocols when PS is excellent [Eastern Cooperative Oncology Group (ECOG) 0-1] and no significant weight loss has occurred because of systemic cancer. A more reduced PS of ECOG 2 or 3 or significant weight loss at diagnosis may lead to more palliative radiotherapy protocols, with symptom control and reduced tumor-related complications being major end points in this setting.

Side Effects of Radiotherapy in the Elderly (Acute and Late)

Three major reviews of interactions between age at presentation and clinical outcome within European Organization for Research and Treatment of Cancer (EORTC) radiotherapy protocols have been performed in 1996, 1997, and 1998. They included 4,406 patients with head and neck, thoracic, and pelvic cancers demonstrating more severe functional acute reactions in older patients (mucositis and sexual dysfunction).

- Elderly patients with lung cancer showed a trend toward increased weight loss following radical radiotherapy.
- Another retrospective analysis of nine EORTC studies in pelvic tumors revealed no differences in acute toxicity between different age groups. Moreover, in most tumor sites, retrospective studies of older patients

have demonstrated no differences in acute and late tolerance to radio-therapy compared with younger ones. In patients with ECOG PS 0 or 1, intensity of acute reactions was similar in older and younger patients. Only duration of recovery from acute reactions seemed to be prolonged (four to seven weeks) in older patients.

- A large review of the EORTC database of head and neck cancers observed no statistically significant difference between age groups in terms of acute and late side effects. But when evaluating age-related differences in toxicities, we have to admit that comprehensive data on chronic toxicities in individual cohorts are currently missing. The overall incidence and severity of all adverse effects seem to be not significantly increased in elderly versus younger ones. Elderly typically experienced longer hospital admission than younger patients, but age was not related to treatment interruption or grade of toxicity.

Specific Side Effects

- With modern radiotherapy techniques, skin reactions are rarely observed unless skin areas lie within the clinical target volume (e.g., in advanced breast cancer).
- Mucosal reactions remain greatly unavoidable (e.g., in head and neck, rectal and prostatic cancer). Healing of mucosal reactions to full recovery occurs at the same kinetics regardless of age. The secondary side effects of mucosal gland reactions are minimized (e.g., in head and neck cancer) by sparing the contralateral side, preventing xerostomia by maintaining functional salivary glands on one side. In prostatic cancer, the organ volumes of bladder, small bowel, and rectal mucosa and the dose administered to these organs can be significantly reduced with modern planning techniques. Higher doses can now be delivered to target volumes in elderly with good or acceptable tolerance.
- There seems to be lesser incidence of radiation-induced nausea/vomiting in the elderly receiving radiotherapy than in younger patients treated with the same protocol. But once nausea/vomiting occurs, the consequences can be worse in elderly who more frequently tend to ignore symptoms of dehydration and develop electrolyte imbalance if not properly supported during radiotherapy courses. In a prospective analysis of radiation-induced gastrointestinal side effects, typically, the frequency of developing nausea/

vomiting was underestimated and thus frequently inadequate and inefficient antiemetic was prescribed. In treatments with high emetic potential (e.g., in abdominal and pelvic cancers) and in concomitant radio-chemotherapy), 5-hydroxytryptamine 3 receptor antagonists should be administered prophylactically rather than symptomatically.

In conclusion, acute and late toxicities have developed at the same percentages amongst all age groups.

Prevention of Side Effects

Novel radiotherapy techniques including external megavoltage radiotherapy (EMRT), conformational intensity-modulated radiotherapy (IMRT), and SRT have benefited from individual 3-D image reconstruction of target volumes and neighboring structures as well as respiratory cycle–gated radiation in organs moving with the respiration cycle ("4-D radiotherapy"). These innovations have allowed individualized calculations of doses delivered to critical organs and optimization of dose delivery. As a result, acute tolerance to radiation in all patients has improved remarkably, whereas incidence and severity of late normal tissue damage have significantly decreased. Such progress has been observed in multiple sites, being of particular relevance for brain, head and neck, thoracic, abdominal, and pelvic malignancies.

The functional reserve of many vital organs typically declines with advancing age, and this alone can cause increased acute toxicity from radiotherapy. Increased damage to normal tissues can be associated with a reduced stem cell reserve in bone marrow as well as in mucosa and with a reduction in the rate of normal tissue cell repopulation. The potential benefit from innovative radiotherapy techniques may be observed in all age groups.

Most of the early literature on increased radiotherapy toxicity in elderly patients stems from series with standard fractionation schedules or non-sophisticated treatment planning. In contrast, reports on age-independent tolerance are based on selected patient populations from clinical trials in high-level institutions. On the basis of positive selection effects (e.g., strict protocol eligibility criteria within prospective trials), these reports may not be totally representative for the overall population. Therefore, the current literature gives biased reports about delivering aggressive treatments within clinical studies that sometimes have to be significantly modified because of acute treatment-related toxicities when given to patients outside clinical trial setting in everyday clinical practice.

Efficacy and Outcome of Radiotherapy in the Aging

Most reports about efficacy of radiotherapy in elderly originate from university hospitals or dedicated cancer centers with specific interest in aggressive approaches. Typically, elderly patients are often per se excluded from clinical trials, and prospective investigations for this selected group are rare. As a consequence, management of cancer in the elderly often cannot be based on first-level evidence.

Population-based data sets from cancer registries may represent alternate ways to gain insight into specific questions within this group. Results in regional and nonuniversity hospitals are typically worse in outcome parameters. Often, radiation therapy in this setting is based on conventional fractionation of only moderate doses. Long-distance transportation to centralized radiotherapy units may be responsible for early discontinuation, significant treatment interruptions, and an increased overall treatment time leading to worse outcome.

To increase overall compliance and delivery in patients, often dose/fractionation compromises by reducing the number of individual fractions and increasing the dose per single fraction are chosen. This hypofractionation approach with fewer than five fractions per week or reduced overall fraction number has been investigated in older and frail patients, leading to overall lower biological doses. The consecutive outcome is generally poorer, at least compared with standard fractionation in most solid tumors. Inadequate doses may potentially compromise the chances of cure for elderly, but instead, the use of novel radiotherapy techniques may significantly improve the quality of life and overall survival in elderly.

There is no clear justification from radiation biology that radiation effects to the tumor tissue itself may be significantly different in older compared with younger patients. When looking at the literature, in fact, subgroup analysis from several randomized trials with concurrent chemoradiotherapy protocols in solid tumors gave even promising results in older patients subset (e.g., Radiation Therapy Oncology Group (RTOG) study 94–10 in locally advanced non-small-cell lung cancer). Therefore, when cure is aimed at, no dose density and overall dose compromises should be allowed for elderly based on their age alone.

Response depends on sensitivity of tumor cells to radiation with adequate tissue oxygenation and ongoing cellular proliferation. The last varies according to the neoplasm site, its histology, and individual tumor biology. Two neoplasms at the same anatomic site and with the same histology may show different response when exposed to the same radiation dose because of differences in proliferation.

- There is little information about the proliferative activity of tumors in the elderly, and there are no clinical data correlating tumor oxygenation with patient age. Experimental data in tumor-bearing mice have demonstrated that oxygenation of tumor cells decreased with age of the tumor-bearing animal. This correlation may be extrapolated to cancer patients, leading to a relevant age-related decrease in tissue perfusion. This, in return, may significantly affect sensitivity of some solid tumors to irradiation. But proliferative activity seems to be inversely correlated with age only for some neoplasms, while in others, it remains independent. In several tumors, the H^3-thymidine labeling index (TLI), a measure of cell proliferation, is decreased in elderly patients, suggesting that sensitivity of tumors to radiation may also be decreased compared with younger ones.
- Tissue hypoxia caused by age-related decrease in circulation and tissue perfusion might lead to reduced tumor sensitivity.

As for local control, there is currently no evidence that solid tumors show different outcomes between different age groups. In a retrospective analysis of nine European EORTC trials in patients with pelvic tumors and age over 70, it was concluded that there were no differences in local control and overall survival following radiotherapy based on patient age. In 1996, 1997, and 1998, three reviews have analyzed the relationship between age at presentation and clinical outcome of patients treated within EORTC radiotherapy protocols. These reviews included 4,406 patients with different cancers [e.g., head and neck, thoracic (including breast and lung cancers), and pelvic cancers (including bladder and prostate)].

- Age did not influence locoregional recurrences and overall survival for head and neck tumors after radical radiotherapy.
- In pelvic malignancies, analysis adjusted for T stage showed comparable local control and disease-free survival between different age

groups for anal, prostate, and uterine cancers. In contrast, younger patients with rectal cancer survived significantly longer than older patients, possibly explained by increased treatment-related mortality in this setting.

On the whole, patient age did not represent a limiting factor for radical radiotherapy in pelvic malignancies excluding rectal cancer.

Palliative Setting: Toxicity and Efficacy Ratio

Once cure is no longer realistic because of large bulky tumors or advanced disease, palliative radiotherapy may still be administered with palliative intent. The predominant aims of radiation in this setting are symptom relief (e.g., bone pain in bone metastases, reduction of neurological symptoms in brain metastases, bleeding of mucosal tumors) and control as well as improvement of quality of life. Toxicity to normal tissues and neighboring organs has to be strongly considered and to be weighted against the overall benefits from palliation. The toxicity:efficacy ratio becomes of major importance, but significant improvements in radiation techniques as outlined above have led to more favorable treatment profiles with a general reduction of toxicity for normal tissues surrounding the tumor.

Curative Setting: Combinations of Chemotherapy and Radiotherapy

Age itself should not hinder curative approaches in the absence of other significant exclusion criteria for aggressive protocols. Biological age and numerical age do not always correspond. Concurrent application of cisplatin-based chemotherapy to radiotherapy significantly improves local control and thus increases the curative potential of treatment in several solid tumors (e.g., lung cancer, head and neck cancer, esophageal cancer, cervical cancer). Within the literature, there are several examples that dosing schedules of reduced individual cisplatin (CDDP) doses (e.g., 6 mg/m^2 CDDP daily application; 20 mg/m^2 CDDP q d_1–d_5; 30 to 50 mg/m^2 CDDP once weekly) may be valuable alternatives and result in significant benefits with regard to overall and long-term survival. Combinations of chemotherapy and radiotherapy may have a significant impact on organ preservation (e.g., rectal cancer, laryngeal cancer, cancer of the floor of the mouth). Therefore, concurrent chemoradiotherapy may be an important alternative to extensive surgical intervention, with underlying higher patient risks in elderly. When deciding on individual treatment protocols in an elderly patient, these alternatives should be acknowledged and discussed within the multimodality team including radiation oncologist, medical oncologist, and preferably also a geriatric physician.

Selection Criteria for Radiotherapy in the Elderly

Comorbidities responsible for impaired organ function in the tumor-bearing region can affect treatment tolerance, may lead to significant side effects or even late complications, and may belong to important patient-related selection factors. Additionally, general (e.g., cardiovascular and pulmonary) comorbidities are significant factors influencing treatment decisions. Increased side effects following radiation in elderly with less tolerance to aggressive treatments are often considered as major contraindications to radiotherapy. Thus, many elderly patients are either not treated at all or treated with reduced intensities because of expected treatment-related toxicities (e.g., radiation mucositis). These increased treatment-related toxicities may be related to significant comorbidities such as chronic cerebrovascular and/or cardiovascular disease, arterial hypertension, diabetes, or significant cardiac, renal, and hepatic dysfunction. However, these comorbidities may differ widely in severity, and even when present in combination, they usually do not implicate a strict contraindication to radiotherapy unless they significantly impact on the overall survival prognosis of the patient compared with the spontaneous course of the disease.

In most patients, comorbidities alone do not justify confining indications of radiotherapy. After correction for physiological and biologic risk factors, a large proportion of elderly patients can still have access to radiation comparable to that in younger ones. However, these considerations are valid for elderly with adequate PS only, and unfortunately, little evidence based on clinical trials and prospective data sets is available yet. Moreover, often at the time of diagnosis, comorbidities are insufficiently controlled. Proper management of comorbidities prior to treatment decision may allow a full-dose radiotherapy delivery even with more aggressive concurrent chemoradiotherapy protocols or application of higher radiation doses alone.

Unfortunately, older patients are less frequently intensively investigated with regard to pulmonary, cardiopulmonary, or vital organ reserve, and as a consequence, they may receive less aggressive therapy based just on general assumption of higher vulnerability to treatment, less tolerance to intensive protocols, and a presumed limited life expectancy.

Another selection criterion for specific patients in everyday clinical practice may be the overall treatment time of radiotherapy. Importantly, some neurological comorbidities like Parkinson's disease or senile dementia can prevent patients from maintaining a reproducible position during treatment over several days and may significantly hamper radiotherapy compliance and tolerance.

Furthermore, the distance between the patient's home and treatment site can be a selection criterion, which may make outpatient treatment difficult. Access to local hosting/housing facilities during treatment period may be unaffordable or even completely unavailable for older patients.

Conclusions

Historically, elderly cancer patients were considered to tolerate aggressive radiation protocols less well based on increased toxicities observed in early clinical trials. Recent improvements in radiotherapy techniques and delivery have significantly reduced side effects, and there is currently no clear evidence for treating elderly patients generally different from younger ones. The available data on normal tissue tolerance to radiotherapy in elderly strongly suggest that those with good functional or PS can tolerate modern schedules comparably well like younger ones. As a consequence, more intensive radiotherapy techniques with curative intent should not be withheld from patients based on their numerical age alone. However, in the individual case, clinically significant comorbidities may sometimes hamper intensive treatment protocols and may lead to decisions for more palliative and less aggressive approaches.

Declaration of Interest:

Dr Eberhardt has not reported any conflicts of interest.

Dr Christoph has not reported any conflicts of interest.

Further Reading

Ausili-Cefaro G, Olmi P. The role of radiotherapy in the management of elderly cancer patients in light of the GROG experience. Crit Rev Oncol Hematol 2001; 39:313–317.

Horiot JC. Radiation therapy and the geriatric oncology patient. J Clin Oncol 2007; 25:1930–1935.

Langer C, Hsu C, Curran WJ, et al. Elderly patients with locally advanced non-small-cell lung cancer benefit from combined-modality therapy: secondary analysis of RTOG 94-10. Proc Am Soc Clin Oncol 2002:21 (abstr 1193).

Momm F, Becker G, Bartelt S, et al. The elderly, fragile tumor patient: radiotherapy as an effective and most feasible treatment modality. J Pain Symptom Manage 2004; 27:3–4.

Montemaggi P, Guerrieri P. Brachytherapy in the elderly. Crit Rev Oncol Hematol 2001; 37:159–167.

Zachariah B, Balducci L. Radiation therapy of the older patient. Hematol Oncol Clin North Am 2000; 14:131–167.

Hormonal Anticancer Treatment in the Senior Cancer Patient

7

B. Seruga, E. Amir, and I.F. Tannock

Division of Hematology and Medical Oncology, Princess Margaret Hospital and University of Toronto, Toronto, Ontario, Canada

Introduction

About 50% of women with breast cancer and ∼70% of men with prostate cancer are diagnosed after the age of 65. Hormonal therapy rarely causes acute side effects and is often recommended in senior patients with breast and prostate cancer. However, hormonal agents are associated with chronic toxicities that can sometimes be life threatening. Thus, before recommending hormonal therapy to elderly patients, the benefits of treatment should be balanced against potential harms and competing risks of morbidity and mortality.

Breast Cancer

In women older than 65 years (and in men with breast cancer), approximately 90% of cancers are estrogen receptor (ER) and/or progesterone receptor (PR) positive.

Hormonal agents used commonly are as follows:

- Selective estrogen receptor modulator (SERM): tamoxifen
- Third-generation aromatase inhibitors (AIs): anastrozole and letrozole (nonsteroidal), and exemestane (steroidal)
- ER downregulator: fulvestrant
- Progestins: megestrol acetate and medroxyprogesterone

(Neo)adjuvant Hormonal Therapy

The Oxford Overview showed that five years of adjuvant tamoxifen reduces the annual rate of death from breast cancer by 31%, including in elderly women. Several phase III clinical trials have evaluated the role of AIs given either up front (e.g., ATAC, BIG 1-98), sequenced/switched after two to three years of tamoxifen (e.g., BIG 1-98, IES, TEAM), or given as extended hormonal therapy after five years of tamoxifen in postmenopausal women with endocrine-responsive breast cancer (e.g., MA.17). Uniformly, these trials demonstrated improved disease-free survival (DFS) rates for AIs compared with tamoxifen, but the benefit is very small in women with low-risk disease. Up-front use of AIs for five years has not demonstrated significant improvement in overall survival as compared with tamoxifen for five years, although there is a small survival benefit from switching strategies. Moreover, at median follow-up of 100 months, there is a worrying excess of deaths with anastrozole as compared with tamoxifen in the ATAC trial.

- An AI should probably be used at some point during adjuvant therapy in older women with intermediate- or high-risk breast cancer, but the optimal use of these agents has not yet been determined. Recent data from the large BIG 1–98 study suggest that five years of treatment with an AI is not superior to a sequenced strategy, which has the advantage of splitting exposure to toxic effects.
- Up-front use of an AI is a reasonable option for postmenopausal women with high-risk breast cancer and in women with contraindications to tamoxifen (e.g., history of thromboembolic disease). There is no basis for continuing AIs beyond five years when used up front or after switching from tamoxifen.
- In selected women with low-risk breast cancer, five years of tamoxifen remains appropriate.
- For postmenopausal women with high-risk disease who completed five years of adjuvant tamoxifen, extended treatment with AIs should be recommended, although data from ongoing studies such as NSABP B42, ABCSG8-SALSA, Dutch Data, GIM4, and SOLE will better determine the optimal duration of endocrine therapy.

In the neoadjuvant setting, randomized clinical trials (e.g., IMPACT and PO24) showed that AIs led to higher rates of response and breast conservation and should be considered in older women with locally advanced breast cancer who have strongly hormone receptor–positive breast cancer and in women with contraindications to chemotherapy (Table 1).

Table I *Role of Hormonal Therapy in Breast Cancer*

Early breast cancer (adjuvant therapy)	
Monotherapy with tamoxifen (5 yr)	■ An option in women with low-risk breast cancer (e.g., small tumor size, N−, and HER-2−) ■ Women who cannot tolerate AIs or have contraindications for their use ■ Men with early breast cancer
Monotherapy with AIs (5 yr)	■ An option in women with high-risk breast cancer (e.g., large tumor size, N+, or HER-2+) ■ Women who cannot tolerate tamoxifen or have contraindications for its use
Sequenced hormonal therapy (AI 2–3 yr after initial use of tamoxifen for 2–3 yr, or vice versa, all together for 5 yr)	■ Women with moderate/high-risk breast cancer, in whom AI was not used up front
Extended hormonal therapy with AI (after 5 yr of tamoxifen)	■ Women with high-risk breast cancer (e.g., N+ disease)
Neoadjuvant hormonal therapy with AIs/tamoxifen (3–4 mo)	■ Women with strongly endocrine-responsive locally advanced breast cancer, especially important for senior women ■ Women with endocrine-responsive breast cancer, in whom chemotherapy is not possible because of contraindications
Advanced breast cancer	
Tamoxifen, non-steroid AIs, steroid AIs, fulvestrant, progestins	■ Sequential administration of available hormonal agents due to incomplete cross-resistance

Abbreviations: AI, aromatase inhibitors; N, lymph node.

Some differences in efficacy between AIs and tamoxifen may be explained by inactivation of, or genetic polymorphism in, the enzyme cytochrome P450 (CYP)2D6, which converts tamoxifen into its active metabolites. Ongoing studies are evaluating the utility of routine testing for genetic polymorphism of CYP2D6. Use of strong and moderate CYP2D6 inhibitors (e.g., the antidepressants fluoxetine, paroxetine, and sertraline) should be discouraged in women who receive tamoxifen; the weak CYP2D6 inhibitors venlafaxine and citalopram are preferred antidepressants in this setting.

Adjuvant therapy with tamoxifen for five years should be recommended to men with early breast cancer. Use of AIs in men has little rationale since 20% of circulating estrogen is produced in the testicles independently of aromatase (Table 1).

Hormonal Therapy in Advanced Breast Cancer

Hormonal therapy is the treatment of choice for older women with meta-static hormone receptor–positive tumors with metastases predominantly to bone and soft tissues and/or with asymptomatic slowly progressive visceral disease. Women with endocrine-responsive breast cancer may benefit from sequential administration of hormonal agents because of incomplete cross-resistance between them: tamoxifen, nonsteroidal AIs, steroidal AIs, progestins, and fulvestrant can be effective.

In randomized clinical trials, AIs demonstrated better response rates and progression-free survival (but not overall survival) as compared with tamoxifen or megestrol acetate. After second-line hormonal treatment, there is no high-level evidence to assist in selecting the optimal agent. When fulvestrant is used after previous hormonal therapies, $\sim 30\%$ of women derive clinical benefit (Table 1).

Women diagnosed with metastatic endocrine-responsive breast cancer who did not receive adjuvant hormonal therapy or had a long disease-free interval after such therapy have a high chance of response to hormonal therapy at the time of recurrence. In contrast, women recurring during adjuvant hormonal therapy have a lower probability of response to further hormonal manipulations.

Although not recommended in the adjuvant setting, AIs can cause protracted stability and objective responses in some men with advanced breast cancer.

False negative determinations of ER and PR status may occur. Thus, hormonal therapy may be active in some women who were reported to have ER-negative and PR-negative tumors, especially in soft tissue and/or bone predominant disease. Further, differences in hormonal status between primary and metastatic sites are reported, and biopsy for determination of hormonal status should be encouraged at time of recurrence.

Side Effects of Hormonal Therapy in Breast Cancer

Major side effects of tamoxifen, AIs, and other hormonal agents used in the treatment of breast cancer are summarized in Table 2. Tamoxifen increases the risk of rare adverse events such as uterine cancer (including uterine sarcoma) and thromboembolic and cerebrovascular disease, and elderly women are at higher risk to develop these toxicities. Women receiving an AI have a lower risk of uterine cancer and thromboembolic or cerebrovascular diseases compared with women on tamoxifen but a higher likelihood of developing arthralgias, fractures, and urogenital atrophy. Bone loss and fractures are of particular concern in older patients, especially those with preexisting osteopenia or osteoporosis: all women receiving an AI should be given calcium and vitamin D supplementation, and their bone density should be assessed annually, with a bisphosphonate prescribed if osteoporosis is documented. Observational data suggest that the prevalence of AI-related joint symptoms is higher than reported in phase III clinical trials. There is no definitive evidence of an increased cardiovascular risk from AIs in relation to placebo despite some increase in comparison with tamoxifen. Side effects can be an important cause of noncompliance with treatment and should therefore be actively sought and addressed during treatment with hormonal therapy.

Prostate Cancer

Prostate cancer is predominantly a disease of older men. In the era of screening with prostate-specific antigen (PSA), most men are diagnosed with localized disease. Senior men with prostate cancer usually die of other causes, with cardiovascular disease being the leading cause of death. In a subset of men with aggressive tumors and without major comorbidity, prostate cancer can rapidly progress to an advanced stage and cause death if not adequately treated.

Table 2 *Major Side Effects of Hormonal Therapy in Breast Cancer*

Tamoxifen	• Hot flashes
	• Venous thromboembolism, stroke
	• Vaginal discharge, uterine hyperplasia/polyps endometrial cancer
	• Fluid retention, muscle cramps
	• Cataract, retinopathy
	• Increased triglycerides (but favorable effect on cholesterol)
	• Other (tumor flare, alopecia, gastrointestinal intolerance, headache)
Aromatase inhibitors	• Hot flashes
	• Vaginal dryness/atrophy
	• Joint pain/stiffness, muscular pain, carpal tunnel syndrome,
	• Bone loss/fracture
	• Other (gastrointestinal intolerance, alopecia, headache, rash, ↑ LFT)
Fulvestrant	• Hot flashes (mild)
	• Gastrointestinal disturbance (mild), ↑ LFT
	• Injection site reaction
	• Other (headache, rash, UTI)
Progestins	• Increased appetite, weight gain
	• Gastrointestinal disturbance
	• Hot flashes
	• Venous thromboembolism
	• Other (tumor flare, rash, gynecomastia, pituitary axis abnormalities)

Abbreviations: ↑ LFT, elevated liver function tests; UTI, urinary tract infection.

The aim of androgen deprivation therapy (ADT) is to deprive prostate cancer of its predominant growth signal: ADT is used increasingly for treatment of prostate cancer, often in spite of evidence showing no effect to prolong overall survival.

Hormonal agents used in men with prostate cancer are as follows:

- Gonadotropin-releasing hormone (GnRH) agonists: goserelin, buserelin leuprolide; alternative is bilateral orchiectomy
- Nonsteroid antiandrogens: bicalutamide, nilutamide, flutamide
- Estrogens: diethylstilbestrol (DES)
- Miscellaneous: ketoconazole, prednisone, dexamethasone
- Experimental: abiraterone acetate, MDV 3100

ADT in Men with Localized and Locally Advanced Prostate Cancer

Decisions regarding treatment should consider the patient's tumor risk, treatment preferences, comorbidity, and life expectancy rather than chronologic age. Depending on the disease status and life expectancy, senior men with localized prostate cancer can be managed with the following treatment options:

- Conservative (watchful waiting or active surveillance)
- Brachytherapy
- External beam radiotherapy
- Radical prostatectomy

Each of these options can be used with or without ADT.

- Randomized clinical trials have demonstrated improved prostate cancer–specific and overall survival from radiation therapy in combination with ADT as compared with radiation therapy alone in men with locally advanced prostate cancer. GnRH agonists should be started before or concurrent with radiotherapy and given for up to three years.
- Use of ADT in combination with brachytherapy or radical prostatectomy has not demonstrated improved overall survival.
  - One small, randomized clinical trial demonstrated that adjuvant ADT after prostatectomy in men with node-positive disease and other high-risk features (e.g., positive margins, involvement of seminal vesicles) might be beneficial, but more evidence is required to support its use in this setting (Table 3).

Table 3 *Role of ADT in Various Clinical Settings of Prostate Cancer*

Localized/locally advanced prostate cancer	
External radiotherapy	In combination with external radiotherapy, ADT improves overall survival in men with locally advanced or intermediate high-risk localized prostate cancer.
Brachytherapy	Neoadjuvant therapy with ADT does not improve overall survival.
Radical prostatectomy	Neoadjuvant ADT does not improve overall survival. Adjuvant ADT in men with no disease does not improve overall survival. Adjuvant ADT in men with N+ disease (and other adverse histopathologic factors such as positive margins, involvement of seminal vesicles) may improve overall survival, but further clinical trials are needed.
No radical local therapy	Primary ADT does not improve overall survival and may be detrimental.
Advanced prostate cancer	
Biochemical (PSA-only) recurrence	No proof from randomized clinical trials that ADT in men with biochemical recurrence is beneficial. However, some men with high risk for cancer-specific death (e.g., Gleason score 8–10, PSA doubling time ≤3 mo) may benefit from immediate ADT.
Asymptomatic metastatic disease	Optimal timing (immediate vs. deferred) of ADT remains controversial. In men who remain asymptomatic for a long time, ADT can be deferred.
Symptomatic prostate cancer	ADT should be given immediately to palliate symptoms and prolong overall survival.

Abbreviations: ADT, androgen deprivation therapy; N, lymph node; PSA, prostate-specific antigen.

Older men are less likely to receive radical treatment for prostate cancer as compared with younger men, but there is a general trend for increasing use of primary ADT. Data from randomized clinical trials and large observational studies show that primary ADT may improve cancer-specific mortality but does not improve overall survival in older men and may even be detrimental (Table 3).

ADT in Advanced Prostate Cancer

To optimize treatment with ADT in senior men with advanced prostate cancer, the following two principles should be followed:

- Monotherapy with a GnRH agonist can be recommended initially. A patient-based meta-analysis in more than 8,000 men demonstrated that addition of an antiandrogen [maximal androgen blockade (MAB)] did not significantly improve overall survival as compared with a GnRH agonist or bilateral orchidectomy alone. Monotherapy is also cheaper and less toxic.
- Intermittent androgen blockade is an option. Results from four randomized clinical trials (one small study published and others reported in meeting abstracts) support noninferiority of intermittent ADT as compared with continuous ADT in men with advanced prostate cancer. The main advantages of intermittent ADT are less time on a potentially toxic therapy, better quality of life, and decreased costs of treatment. However, all but one of the randomized clinical trials evaluated MAB, which cannot be considered standard of care, and future clinical trials should address intermittent versus continuous monotherapy.

Biochemical Relapse

Every third man after radical prostatectomy or radiotherapy experiences biochemical (PSA-only) relapse: only a subset of them will develop overt metastases, and an even smaller subset will die of prostate cancer. Radiation therapy is the only potentially curative therapy for men with biochemical recurrence after radical prostatectomy. ADT is not curative, and there is no evidence from randomized clinical trials to support its use in men with biochemical recurrence. It is reasonable to consider treatment with ADT only in a subgroup of men with a high risk for cancer-specific death (e.g., PSA doubling time ≤ 3 months, Gleason score 8–10, and short time from primary local treatment to the development of recurrence) (Table 3).

Metastatic Prostate Cancer

Men with symptomatic metastatic prostate cancer should be treated with ADT. However, many men with metastases diagnosed by computer tomography or bone scan remain asymptomatic for a long time: it is reasonable to offer ADT to men with asymptomatic metastatic disease and rapidly rising PSA but not to those with slow progression.

Initially, more than 80% of patients respond to GnRH agonists or bilateral orchidectomy, but their disease will eventually progress after a median of 18 to 20 months. At progression, about one-third of men respond to the addition of an antiandrogen, and about 10% to 20% of those patients who respond and then progress will respond to withdrawal of the antiandrogen. Some men may respond to further hormonal therapies including dexamethasone, ketoconazole, or estrogen (Table 3); their activity can be explained by (*i*) suppressed production of adrenal androgens (e.g., ketoconazole and dexamethasone) and (*ii*) direct anticancer effects (e.g., estrogens and dexamethasone).

Promising new agents include abiraterone acetate, which blocks production of adrenal androgens by the inhibition of the CYP17A1 enzyme and MDV 3100, which is a new-generation potent antiandrogen. Both drugs show promising activity in early-phase clinical trials and are being evaluated in phase III trials.

Side Effects of ADT

The risk of treatment with GnRH analogues needs to be assessed carefully in older men with prostate cancer. Well-recognized side effects include hot flashes, muscle loss, anemia, sexual dysfunction, and gynecomastia, all of which can decrease quality of life. ADT can also increase risk for more serious and potentially life-threatening side effects such as metabolic syndrome, cardiovascular disease, and bone fractures. These toxicities can appear after a short period (e.g., months) of therapy with GnRH agonists and are particularly salient for a senior population. All men receiving ADT should receive calcium and vitamin D supplementation and should have evaluation of bone density periodically; annual treatment with zoledronic acid can prevent bone loss in those at risk. Health professionals should also evaluate cardiovascular risk when prescribing ADT to senior men with prostate cancer, especially in settings without compelling evidence for its use (Table 4).

Table 4 *Major Side Effects of Androgen Deprivation Therapy*

GnRH agonists	■ Male menopausal symptoms
	■ Muscle loss
	■ Bone loss/fractures
	■ Loss of libido, impotence, gynecomastia
	■ Metabolic syndrome, diabetes, cardiovascular disease
	■ Anemia
Antiandrogens (major drug-specific side effects)	■ Male menopausal symptoms
	■ Gastrointestinal disturbance (bicalutamide, flutamide)
	■ Gynecomastia/mastodynia (bicalutamide)
	■ Occular toxicity (nilutamide)
	■ Pulmonary toxicity (nilutamide)
Miscellaneous	■ Cardiovascular disease (estrogens)
	■ Liver toxicity, gastrointestinal disturbance (ketoconazole)
	■ Dermatologic toxicity (ketoconazole)
	■ Diabetes (prednisone)
	■ Hypertension (prednisone)

Abbreviation: GnRH, gonadotropin-releasing hormone.

Declaration of Interest:

Dr Tannock has reported that he advises a number of companies including Sanofi-Aventis about clinical trials for prostate cancer, for which he receives donations for his research fund. He does not accept personal remuneration from companies.

Dr Seruga has reported no conflicts of interest.

Dr Amir has reported that he is on the advisory board for AstraZeneca Canada and received honoraria from AstraZeneca.

Further Reading

Seruga B, Tannock IF. Up-front use of aromatase inhibitors as adjuvant therapy for breast cancer: the emperor has no clothes. J Clin Oncol 2009; 27:2566–2567.

Cytotoxic and Targeted Anticancer Treatment in the Senior Cancer Patient

H. Wildiers

Department of General Medical Oncology/Multidisciplinary Breast Centre,
University Hospitals Leuven, Leuven, Belgium

Introduction

Systemic anticancer therapy is a mainstay in the fight against cancer. Chemotherapy is highly effective in attacking tumor cells spread all over the body. However, chemotherapy is sometimes related with significant toxicity.

- In some settings such as large-cell non-Hodgkin lymphoma (NHL), the benefits of chemotherapy are generally much larger than the potential side effects.
- In other settings such as in many metastatic solid tumors, the absolute benefits are less extensive, and side effects and quality of life are of utmost importance.

In senior individuals, the potential of harming patients with chemotherapy is even higher than that in the younger population. It is hoped that the upcoming targeted therapies have a better therapeutic index and can be more beneficial in older cancer patients. However, clinical experience shows that caution is also warranted with targeted therapy in older patients.

Chemotherapy in Senior Adults

Indications

In principle, the same indications for chemotherapy are present in older and younger cancer patients. Specific concerns can be present however.

- In *curative* settings, such as treatment of NHL, chemotherapy dose intensity is crucial. NHL is aggressive with very poor prognosis if untreated. Soft/low-dose regimens have been shown to be clearly inferior to standard therapy.
- In *adjuvant* settings of solid tumors, such as colorectal and breast cancer, the absolute benefits of chemotherapy are usually rather small and generally limited to 5% to 10% of patients, while all patients are exposed to potential toxicity. Moreover, the risks of chemotherapy increase with age, such as the risk of myelosuppression or cardiac failure with anthracyclines. It has also been shown that lowering the dose or dose intensity or choosing "soft" chemotherapy such as capecitabine for breast cancer is clearly inferior to standard therapy. The decision of giving adjuvant chemotherapy is thus a delicate decision integrating the absolute risk of recurrence (based on tumor characteristics) and based on patients characteristics such as life expectancy, comorbidity, and the patient's desire. If the decision is made, adequate dosing and regimens are warranted.
- In *metastatic* settings of solid tumors, the goal is palliation and tumor control without causing excessive toxicity. Chemotherapy can be helpful, but continuous monitoring is required to evaluate whether toxicity is not taking the upper hand.

Considerations in the Use of Chemotherapy in Older Individuals

If the decision for giving chemotherapy is made, it is important to keep in mind some specific age-related aspects summarized in Tables 1 to 3.

Side Effects in Older Individuals

Elderly patients have a decreased tolerance to chemotherapy in general, with increased incidence of various toxicities. Some side effects are rather drug specific, such as cardiac failure and anthracyclines, or neuropathy and taxanes/cisplatin.

- Myelosuppression is a more general side effect and is the major dose-limiting toxicity of many modern chemotherapeutic drugs. Initial retrospective analyses of data from clinical trials in patients with solid tumors showed no correlation between age and myelosuppression.

Table 1 Considerations When Using Chemotherapy in Senior Individuals

Treatment individualization	Senior adults are the utmost example of heterogeneity, and adaptation to the individual situation is always required.
Geriatric assessment	Geriatric assessment is the best way to obtain a more global view on the general health situation of the patient and is advised in all cancer patients ≥ 70 years of age.
Supportive or protective agents	Antiemetics, growth factors, pain killers, and antidiarrheal drugs can be crucial to continue treatment.
Risk of drug interactions	Polypharmacy is frequent in senior adults, and there is a great risk for drug interactions and potentially increased toxicity.
Compliance	Compliance can be an important issue undermining the efficacy of chemotherapy (mainly for oral cytostatics) or potentially increasing toxicity (if supportive drugs are not taken appropriately at home).
Possibility of less toxic therapy	There might be good alternatives in some situations for chemotherapy, such as hormonal therapies, local radiotherapy, or surgery for localized problems.
Maintain adequate hydration	Elderly patients have a tendency to drink less, especially when feeling ill, and are more intolerant of dehydration. Poor hydration can lead to decreased clearance and increased toxicity, especially for drugs subject to renal excretion.
Define the aim of chemotherapy	It is crucial to realize why chemotherapy is given. The need for maintaining dose and dose intensity can be very different depending on the setting.
Renal function	Renal function declines continuously with aging, and comorbidity can even further compromise renal function in the elderly. Moreover, a large part of cytostatic drugs are renally excreted. If renal function declines and the same dose of chemotherapy is given, global exposition [e.g., as defined by

(Continued)

Table 1 Considerations When Using Chemotherapy in Senior Individuals (Continued)

	area under the curve (AUC)] can markedly increase with accompanying increased toxicity. Dose adaptation, according to renal function, is thus mandatory to avoid excessive toxicity. The International Society of Geriatric Oncology (SIOG) has made specific guidelines on the determination of renal function in elderly, as well on dose adaptation of specific chemotherapeutic agents in renal dysfunction.
Be aware of pharmacological and clinical data for specific chemotherapy drugs	For most classical chemotherapeutic drugs, at least some data are available on age-related pharmacokinetics and dosing (see also Tables 2 and 3). Oncologists should be aware of these data, and take them into account when prescribing chemotherapy to older individuals. However, it should be stated that dose adaptation based on age-related pharmacological changes is an unvalidated approach since clinical trials prospectively testing the efficacy and toxicity of age-related dose adaptation versus standard dosing are lacking.

Severe selection bias was present in these studies however, limiting the generalization of these conclusions to the whole geriatric population. More recent data clearly show that the risk of neutropenia increases with age, for instance, in NHL or breast cancer. Because of the increased risk of neutropenia and related complications in senior adults, and the potential for better outcomes when maintaining dose intensity in certain settings, prophylaxis with a colony-stimulating factor starting in the first cycle should be considered in elderly patients.

- Mucositis (intestinal and/or oral) is a common side effect of several chemotherapeutic drugs, for example, irinotecan and 5-fluorouracil. Older persons seem to be more susceptible to this side effect, and aggressive and effective management of these and other side effects is crucial in senior adults.

Table 2   *Pharmacokinetic Parameters That Might Change with Aging and Might Influence Efficacy/Toxicity of Chemotherapy*

Parameter changes	Clinical consequences
Absorption: decreased	Oral chemotherapy (e.g., capecitabine) might be less effective in elderly.
Volume of distribution: decreased	Serum concentrations and toxicity of several chemotherapeutics might increase (e.g., cisplatin, taxanes, etoposide, irinotecan).
Hepatic metabolism: decreased	Not well known, may affect serum concentrations of chemotherapeutics eliminated by hepatic metabolism (e.g., taxanes, cyclophosphamide, anthracyclines).
Renal excretion: decreased	Dosing should be adapted to present recommendations to avoid excessive serum concentrations and toxicity from renally excreted chemotherapeutics (e.g., carboplatin, topotecan, methotrexate).

Source: Courtesy of Elsevier.

Targeted Therapies in Senior Adults

Targeted therapies do not induce classical side effects of chemotherapy in general (e.g., hair loss, deep neutropenia, nausea, and vomiting) and are certainly promising for elderly individuals, but care is warranted since specific side effects might also occur.

- In HER-2/neu-positive breast cancer, trastuzumab was the first modern "targeted therapy" established with a favorable safety profile. However, age was a documented risk factor for congestive heart failure in patients receiving trastuzumab but depends probably more on preexisting comorbidities than on age by itself.
- Angiogenesis inhibitors can cause thrombosis and hypertension, and age is an important risk factor.

Table 3 *Age-Related Effects on Pharmacokinetics of Frequently Used Chemotherapeutics and Consequences*

Alkylating agents
- *Cyclophosphamide*
  - PK not different, some increased toxicity on PD.
  - Important liver metabolism, effect of age-related decrease in hepatic function is unknown.
  - Adapt to renal function.
  - No arguments for a priori dose reduction in elderly.
- *Cisplatin*
  - Increased AUC and toxicity in elderly.
  - Adapt to renal function.
  - Consider the lower range of dosage (e.g., 60 mg/m^2) and preferably at a reduced infusion rate (e.g., over 24 hr).
- *Carboplatin*
  - Adapt to renal function (Calvert formula).
- *Oxaliplatin*
  - No arguments for a priori dose reduction in elderly.

Taxanes
- *Paclitaxel*
  - Conflicting PK data on paclitaxel clearance in elderly.
  - Several trials show feasibility of both every-three-week and weekly paclitaxel in elderly patients.
  - No arguments for a priori dose reduction in elderly.
- *Docetaxel*
  - Docetaxel PK is only minimally influenced by age.
  - Elderly patients are somewhat more vulnerable to side effects, but as for PK, interpatient variability is larger than age-related variability.
  - In principal, standard regimens of docetaxel can be used (dose and schedule depend on clinical setting), but high dose needs to be given with caution.

(Continued)

Table 3 *Age-Related Effects on Pharmacokinetics of Frequently Used Chemotherapeutics and Consequences (Continued)*

Topo-isomerase inhibitors
- *Etoposide* (topo II)
  - High variability in oral absorption.
  - Increased AUC and toxicity in elderly.
  - Dose adaptation according to albumin, bilirubin, and renal function should be considered.
- *Irinotecan* (topo I)
  - Increased AUC and diarrhea in elderly.
  - A lower dose (e.g., 300 mg/m^2 q3w instead of 350 mg/m^2 q3w) could be considered for $\geq$age 70.
- *Topotecan* (topo I)
  - Adapt to renal function.
  - Consider weekly regimens (less myelosuppression).

Antimetabolites
- *Methotrexate*
  - AUC possibly increased.
  - Adapt to renal function.
- *Fluorouracil*
  - PK and toxicity not majorly influenced.
- *Capecitabine*
  - Lower dose such as 1000 mg/m^2 bid instead of 1250 mg/m^2 seems equally effective with less side effects.
  - Adapt to renal function.
- *Gemcitabine*
  - Unpredictable PK.
  - Generally good tolerance in elderly.

Antitumor antibiotics
- *Doxorubicin*
  - Increased peak plasma concentrations.
  - Increased myelosuppression and cardiotoxicity.

(Continued)

Table 3 *Age-Related Effects on Pharmacokinetics of Frequently Used Chemotherapeutics and Consequences (Continued)*

◦ At full dose (e.g., CHOP, AC) relatively toxic.
◦ Possible solutions.
   – Dose reduction if being given in palliative setting
   – Alternative administration regimens: e.g., weekly
   – Liposomal forms
   – Removal of doxorubicin in lymphoma regimens
   – Growth factors

Abbreviations: PK, pharmacokinetics; AUC, area under the curve; PD, pharmacodynamics; CHOP, cyclophosphamide, doxorubicin, vincristine, and prednisone; AC, doxorubicin and cyclophosphamide.
Source: Courtesy of Elsevier.

◦ For instance, a pooled analysis of bevacizumab-treated patients with all types of cancer from five randomized trials demonstrated that patients >age 65 are at increased risk of arterial thromboembolic events, particularly when bevacizumab was given in combination with chemotherapy.
◦ With small-molecule tyrosine kinase inhibitors of angiogenesis, a high incidence of cardiac failure has been demonstrated and is of great concern for the senior population that often has cardiac comorbidity.

A major problem is that most clinical trials only include "healthy" senior patients, so results and toxicity data cannot be extrapolated to the general senior population. It is crucial that upcoming targeted therapies are also studied in senior patients to establish the safety and efficacy in that particular population.

Declaration of Interest:

Dr Wildiers has reported no conflicts of interest.

Further Reading

Lichtman SM, Wildiers H, Chatelut E, et al. International Society of Geriatric Oncology chemotherapy taskforce: evaluation of chemotherapy in older patients—an analysis of the medical literature. J Clin Oncol 2007; 25:1832–1843.

Lichtman SM, Wildiers H, Launay-Vacher V, et al. International Society of Geriatric Oncology (SIOG) recommendations for the adjustment of dosing in elderly cancer patients with renal insufficiency. Eur J Cancer 2007; 43:14–34.

Wildiers H. Mastering chemotherapy dose reduction in elderly cancer patients. Eur J Cancer 2007; 43:2235–2241.

Wildiers H, Highley MS, De Bruijn EA, et al. Pharmacology of anticancer drugs in the elderly population. Clin Pharmacokinet 2003; 42:1213–1242.

Treatment of Lymphoma in the Elderly Population

9

A.S. Michallet and B. Coiffier

Hospices civils de Lyon, Service d'Hématologie Clinique,
Pierre Benite, France

Introduction

Life expectancy has increased impressively over the past century; this has naturally resulted in an increase in the number of older patients. Non-Hodgkin lymphoma is especially relevant in the elderly patient population as the median age of patients with this disorder is 65 years. All lymphoma subtypes are observed in this population, with some modest differences compared with those encountered in younger patients. Most of the large epidemiologic studies have found that elderly patients have a higher percentage of patients with aggressive lymphomas (diffuse large B-cell lymphoma, peripheral T-cell and less frequently anaplastic large cell lymphoma, Burkitt's lymphomas). No specific chromosomal or genetic features have been described in elderly patients.

Diagnosis and Prognosis

Clinical and biological characteristics at presentation are similar to those observed in younger patients. Staging at diagnosis is similar with clinical examination, computed tomography (CT) scan and if possible positron emission tomography (PET) scan, bone marrow biopsy, serum lactate dehydrogenase (LDH), serum β2-microglobulin, human immunodeficiency virus (HIV), and hepatitis B serologies.

Particular attention must be given to the presence of comorbidities [cumulative illness rating score (CIRS)] and their functional effect.

To assess therapeutic options, the international prognostic index (IPI) better describes prognosis than stage for older patients. The IPI includes items that reflect the host status [age, performance status (PS)] as well as the extent of the disease (disease stage, LDH level, and number of extranodal disease sites). For younger or older patients, a simplified index, the age-adjusted IPI, which only uses stage, PS, and LDH level, may be used to estimate the risk of failure. In older patients, determination of the PS is the most subjective criterion.

Another element to take into account for determining the treatment is the complexity and the heterogeneity of this elderly population. Presence of other diseases, organ dysfunction, and polymedications are factors that can compromise the ability to tolerate therapy. A variety of new methods [comprehensive geriatric assessement (CGA), CIRS] are actually being evaluated to predict prognosis and to select the appropriate population that could receive a curative therapy.

Older patients often have a decrease in the glomerular filtration rate and a delay in drug excretion such that drug doses may have to be tailored to creatinine clearance.

Furthermore, the decrease of the liver function could alter the metabolism of a lot of drugs. A multidisciplinary approach with geriatric evaluation is essential to define the specific therapy (Fig. 1).

In the elderly, hematopoietic reserve capacity is often altered. Because of myelotoxicity, the risk of febrile neutropenia and infectious complications are increased in older patients treated with curative strategy. The American

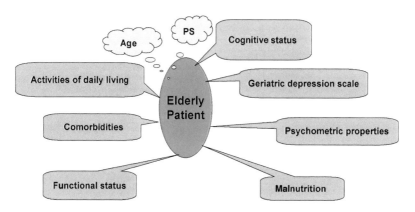

Figure 1 Complexity of the elderly population.

Society of Clinical Oncology and the European Organization for Research and Treatment of Cancer have developed guidelines to the use of supportive care like granulocyte colony-stimulating factor (G-CSF) and erythropoietin-stimulating agents (ESA) to prevent these complications. Both societies have considered age as an increased risk of infectious complications and recommended the systematic use of G-CSF for older patients when the risk of neutropenia is more than 20%.

Furthermore, older patients have reduced emotional tolerance considering the invasive procedures. It is then essential to propose an integrated approach where the physician explains the objectives of the treatment with a curative or palliative option and where the patient and his family take an active role in the therapeutic project.

Treatment

Considering all of these elements in the elderly population, two approaches can be proposed for the first-line treatment of diffuse large B-cell lymphomas.

The first approach uses the same treatments as in younger patients, and the second one prioritizes quality of life and uses less toxic but less effective treatments and can be considered as a palliative approach (Fig. 2). This debate is essential in case of diffuse large B-cell lymphoma because this lymphoma is potentially curable. Its therapy has undergone a renaissance 10 years ago with the addition of rituximab to standard regimens, such as cyclophosphamide, doxorubicin, vincristine, and prednisone (CHOP). Several large phase III studies have compared the CHOP regimen and rituximab-CHOP (R-CHOP) regimen, including three studies confined to the elderly patient population. The addition of rituximab results in an improved outcome, with higher response rates and prolongation of survival (progression-free survival, disease-free survival, and overall survival). Furthermore, the R-CHOP regimen achieves similar progression-free survival with what is observed in a younger population, confirming the high correlation between the quality of response and the duration of the survival irrespective of patient age. The German Lymphoma Study Group has shown that results may be improved when the CHOP regimen, CHOP-14, is given every two weeks compared with the classical every-three-weeks schedule. However, recent comparative studies did not confirm this observation.

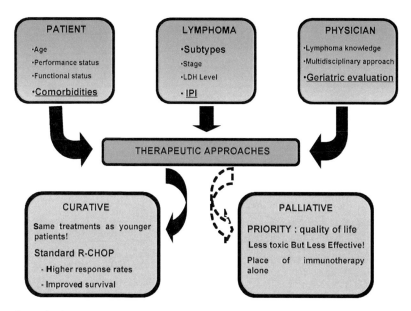

Figure 2 Integrated approach to assess therapeutic options in older patients with lymphomas.

The current conclusion is that R-CHOP is recommended for the treatment of older patients with diffuse large B-cell lymphomas except for patients with cardiac comorbidity. In fact, nonfit patients with altered cardiac function because of decrease in ventricular ejection rate or other diseases are not able to tolerate R-CHOP. In this case, a combination of rituximab with ifosfamide and etoposide is frequently used with good results.

For patients older than 80, very few studies have been reported. For the most fit of them, a standard R-CHOP or a low-dose R-CHOP (mini-R-CHOP) is the recommended treatment.

At time of relapse, the prognosis is very poor, with few therapeutic possibilities. Several salvage regimens can be used, but cisplatin-containing regimens are frequently contraindicated because of the renal dysfunction often associated with age. Whatever regimen is used, median survival is usually around six months, and the best therapeutic option is possibly a palliative approach favoring a highest quality of life over the duration of survival. However, a subgroup of patients younger than 70 years and medically fit could be candidates to highest-dose salvage and autologous stem cell transplantation.

Another strategy for relapsing older patients is the use of novel agents alone or combined with classical chemotherapy. Antiangiogenic agents, such as thalidomide or lenalidomide, have proven to be efficient and could be an option in progressive disease.

Finally, concerning the therapeutic strategies for indolent lymphomas, the watch-and-wait strategy may be applied to most of these patients. When treatment is needed, those used for younger patients are the best choice.

Conclusions

Age appears to be an adverse prognostic factor for survival of patients with lymphoma, particularly the aggressive subtypes, because physicians usually decrease the dose of drugs. The best way to improve survival of the elderly population is to treat them with an optimal chemotherapy and a curative approach.

Declaration of Interest:

Prof Coiffier has reported that he is currently conducting research with Roche, Celgene, Sanofi, GSK, Pfizer and Millenium. He is also a member of the speaker's bureau of Roche, Amgen, GSK and Celgene.

Dr Michallet has reported no conflicts of interest.

Further Reading

Aapro MS, Cameron DA, Pettengell R, et al. EORTC guidelines for the use of granulocyte-colony stimulating factor to reduce the incidence of chemotherapy-induced febrile neutropenia in adult patients with lymphomas and solid tumors. Eur J Cancer 2006; 42:2433–2453.

Coiffier B, Lepage E, Briere J, et al. CHOP chemotherapy plus rituximab compared with CHOP alone in elderly patients with diffuse large B-cell lymphoma. N Engl J Med 2002; 346:235–242.

Extermann M, Aapro MS, Bernabei R, et al. Use of comprehensive geriatric assessment in older cancer patients: Recommendations from the task force on

CGA of the International Society of Geriatric Oncology (SIOG). Crit Rev Oncol Hematol 2005; 55:241–252.

Feugier P, Van Hoof A, Sebban C, et al. Long-term results of the R-CHOP study in the treatment of elderly patients with diffuse large B-cell lymphoma: a study by he Groupe d'Etude des Lymphomes de l'Adulte. J Clin Oncol 2005; 23:4117–4126.

Jantunen E. Autologous stem cell transplantation beyond 60 years of age. Bone Marrow Transplant 2006; 38:715–720.

Pfreundschuch M, Schubert J, Ziepert M, et al. Six versus eight cycles of bi-weekly CHOP-14 with or without rituximab in elderly patients with aggressive CD20+ B-cell lymphomas: a randomised controlled trial (RICOVER-60). Lancet Oncol 2008; 9:105–116.

Weisenburger DD. Epidemiology of non-Hodgkin's lymphoma: recent findings regarding en emerging epidemic. Ann Oncol 1994; 5:19–24.

Westin E, Longo D. Lymphoma and myeloma in older patients. Semin Oncol 2004; 31:198–205.

Management of Myeloproliferative Diseases in Senior Patients

D. Wolf and R. Stauder

Department of Internal Medicine V, Hematology and Oncology, Innsbruck Medical University, Innsbruck, Austria

Diagnosis and Classification of Myeloproliferative Disorders

Myeloproliferative disorders (MPD) are relatively rare chronic hematologic malignancies that include the classic MPD: the Philadelphia chromosome (PH)-negative essential thrombocythemia (ET), primary myelofibrosis (PMF) and polycythemia vera (PV) and Philadelphia chromosome-positive chronic myelogenous leukemia (CML). Atypical MPD include molecularly defined platelet-derived growth factor (PDGFR) A—rearranged eosinophilic/mast cell disorders; PDGFR B—rearranged eosinophilic disorders; systemic mastocytosis associated with c-kit mutation; 8p11 myeloproliferative syndrome; and juvenile myelomonocytic leukemia with recurrent mutations of RAS.

PH-negative MPD are usually diagnosed later in life, at an average median age of 60, which is also the median age of CML diagnosis. Thus, a considerable proportion of this patient group is above 60 years at diagnosis including a relevant proportion reaching the age of senior patients, that is, 70+ years. Moreover, when considering the fact that the median survival of patients with MPD is relatively long, the prevalence of elderly patients with MPD is high. Despite this clinical reality, specific treatment considerations in the era of targeted therapies in this particular patient population have rarely been addressed in clinical trials.

Independent of patients' age, MPD are classified according to the revised World Health Organization (WHO) classification since 2008 (Table 1). The

Table 1 *Diagnostic Criteria for Myeloproliferative Disorders According to the Revised World Health Organization*

Criteria	CML	ET	PV	PMF
Major	1. BM biopsy showing hyperplasia of myelopoiesis and megakaryopoiesis. 2. Detection of Philadelphia chromosome by conventional cytogenetics and by FISH 3. Detection of the BCR-ABL fusion transcript by PCR	1. Sustained platelet count ≥450 × 109/L during workup period 2. BM biopsy showing proliferation mainly of the megakaryocytic lineage with increased numbers of enlarged, mature megakaryocytes; no significant increase or left shift of neutrophil granulopoiesis or erythropoiesis 3. Not meeting WHO criteria for PV, PMF, CML, MDS, or other myeloid neoplasm	1. Hemoglobin >18.5 g/dL in men, 16.5 g/dL in women, or other evidence of increased red cell volume 2. Presence of JAK2617V > F or other functionally similar mutation such as JAK2 exon 12 mutation	1. Presence of megakaryocyte proliferation and atypia, usually accompanied by either reticulin and/or collagen fibrosis, or in the absence of significant reticulin fibrosis, the megakaryocyte changes must be accompanied by an increased BM cellularity characterized by granulocytic proliferation and often decreased erythropoiesis (i.e., prefibrotic cellular-phase disease)

(Continued)

Criteria	CML	ET	PV	PMF
		4. Demonstration of JAK2617V > F or other clonal marker or, in the absence of a clonal marker, no evidence for reactive thrombocytosis		2. Not meeting WHO criteria for PV, PMF, CML, MDS, or other myeloid neoplasm 3. Demonstration of JAK2617V > F or other clonal marker (e.g., MPL515W>L/K), or in the absence of a clonal marker, no evidence of BM fibrosis due to underlying inflammatory or other neoplastic diseases
Minor			1. BM biopsy showing hypercellularity for age with trilineage growth	1. Leukoerythroblastosis 2. Increase in serum lactate dehydrogenase level

(panmyelosis) with prominent erythroid, granulocytic, and megakaryocytic proliferation

2. Serum erythropoietin level below the reference range for normal
3. Endogenous erythroid colony formation in vitro

3. Anemia
4. Palpable splenomegaly

For diagnosis of PV: The presence of both major and one minor criteria or the presence of the first major criterion together with two minor criteria is required.
For diagnosis of ET: All four major criteria are required.
For diagnosis of PMF: Diagnosis requires meeting all three major criteria and two minor criteria.
Abbreviations: BM: bone marrow; FISH: fluorescence in situ hybridization; PCR: polymerase chain reaction; WHO: World Health Organization.

required diagnostic procedures can be deduced from these criteria: physical examination, examination of a blood sample, a bone marrow biopsy, as well as molecular biology [including analysis of classical cytogenetics, fluorescence in situ hybridization (FISH) for detection of the Philadelphia chromosome, and mutation analysis for diagnosis of JAK-2]. An enlarged spleen is often detected by physical examination, but ultrasound or computed tomography scans may occasionally be necessary.

Treatment Strategies of MPD in the Senior Patient
Chronic Myeloid Leukemia

Preliminary observations indicate that elderly CML patients are less frequently treated with the current standard first-line therapy, that is, 400 mg of the tyrosine kinase inhibitor imatinib once daily. Recent data from large multicenter studies from the German CML study group as well as the Italian GIMEMA CML Working Party have addressed this particular issue.

Efficacy of Imatinib in Senior Patients

Both studies compared patients enrolled in phase III trials below 65 versus patients ≥65 years. The median daily dose was not different between both groups. In the German CML study IV, older patients achieved complete cytogenetic responses (CCR) and major molecular responses significantly later than younger patients (12.3 vs. 10.7 months and 24.1 vs. 15.9 months, respectively). In contrast, the Italian cooperative group (which also included patients receiving 800 mg daily, which is not the standard dose) was not able to detect statistical significant differences in response rates between young and elderly CML patients (cumulative CCR rate 88% vs. 84% and 82% vs. 81%, respectively). The rate of treatment failures according to the European LeukemiaNet (ELN) guidelines, as well as progression rates and rate of CML-related deaths were also comparable.

Toxicity of Imatinib in Senior Patients

In the German trial, a higher proportion of older patients discontinued treatment (12.4% vs. 8.4%). Various differences were observed in the profile of grade III/IV adverse events (AEs). Hematologic AEs were more common in the older as compared with the younger patient cohort (leu-kopenia <2000 leukocytes/μl 4.2% vs. 2.8% and thrombocytopenia <50000/μl 4.2% vs. 2.8%, respectively). Most nonhematologic AEs were not different between the two age groups (gastrointestinal 29% vs. 28%, myalgia 17% vs. 16%). Edema and neurological symptoms were even higher in younger than in older patients (17% vs. 23% and 6% vs. 15%, respectively), whereas dermatologic side effects were more frequent in the older patient population (17% vs. 13%).

Polythemia Vera

In PV the increased number of red blood cells or platelets can cause bleeding problems and induce clot formation in blood vessels. This can cause serious complications such as stroke or heart attack. In patients older than 65 years, the risk of stroke and heart attack is higher, and PV is more likely to transform into acute leukemia or PMF. Without treatment, patients with PV usually die from bleeding or blood clotting within months. In contrast, median survival is about 10 years in older patients under appro-priate therapy. Many patients can reach their normal life expectancy if they do not develop marrow fibrosis or leukemia.

Currently, there are no studies available specifically addressing the ques-tion how senior PV patients should be treated. However, the treatment options currently available for this disease are generally well tolerated and can, after careful evaluation of relevant comorbidities of the individual patient, be also applied to elderly patients.

- Periodically removing erythrocytes by phlebotomy represents a safe and very effective way to treat low-risk PV patients. The hematocrit should be kept below 45% in men and 43% in women.
- Because of platelet activation, low-risk patients should also receive low-dose aspirin (i.e., 100 mg per day), which can also be easily applied (major side effects are gastrointestinal intolerance and bleeding) in elderly patients who have no contraindications against aspirin.
- Patients with a higher risk of clotting (i.e., having risk factors such as leukocytosis, age >65 years, and/or a previous thrombotic event) should be treated with cytotoxic agents, such as hydroxyurea. This drug has relatively few side effects, and its beneficial effects in terms of prevention of vascular complications outweigh its potential harm (i.e.,

induction of leukemia), which may not be as relevant in the elderly population when compared with younger patients.

- In the case of insufficient response to hydroxyurea, interferon-α or anagrelide (especially when thrombocytosis is present) can be suggested. Interferon-α may be particularly difficult to tolerate as its side effects include flu-like symptoms (e.g., fever, chills, postnasal drip, and poor appetite), fatigue, weight loss, depression, insomnia, memory loss, and nausea.

- Finally, radioactive phosphorus still represents a valuable option for elderly patients who are unable to take oral medication or who are not expected to need many years of treatment. In 80% to 90% of patients, this treatment can suppress the disease symptoms for months up to several years.

Among the most difficult complications to treat is splenomegaly, which can often be controlled by phlebotomy in early-stage disease, but later on other treatment modalities, such as hydroxyurea, or surgical removal may be necessary. Radiation treatments directed at the spleen may be another option, but the bone marrow reserve has to be determined before by bone marrow biopsy, as marrow function might be significantly suppressed by this procedure.

Essential Thrombocytosis

In ET, the increased number of platelets in the blood can cause thrombotic and hemorrhagic complications. Currently, no randomized clinical studies are available that can provide the optimal point for treatment initiation. However, the number of thrombocytes, age, history of thromboembolic complications, and vascular risk factors allow a risk categorization, which then prompts treatment initiation.

Platelet-lowering treatment is indicated for patients over 60 years of age or with platelet counts over $1.5 \times 10^6/\mu L$ or either bleeding or thromboembolic complications associated with ET.

- Hydroxyurea results in a reduction in the incidence of total arterial thrombosis when compared with anagrelide or with no treatment. However, no effect of hydroxyurea has been shown for stroke, myocardial infarction, or overall survival.

- Anagrelide is inferior to hydroxyurea in controlling arterial thrombosis, and its efficacy in comparison with no cytoreductive therapy has not been established. Although venous thrombosis was reduced in the anagrelide arm of the study comparing anagrelide with aspirin with hydroxyurea with aspirin, it is unclear whether the rate is increased by hydroxyurea or decreased by anagrelide. Notably, serious bleeding is increased with anagrelide in combination with aspirin, thus, this combination should be avoided.

Because of the fact that age >60 years is a major risk factor for thrombosis or bleeding events, all senior patients should be treated with cytoreductive treatment. Treatment decision includes careful evaluation or relevant comorbidities to prevent treatment-related side effects (i.e., advanced renal insufficiency and chronic heart failure are relative contraindications for anagrelide).

Primary Myelofibrosis

Currently, despite allogeneic stem cell transplantation, which is, in principle, only applicable to patients <65 years of age with a suitable donor, no curative treatment option is available for patients with PMF. Studies specifically addressing the question of the optimal treatment strategy in elderly patients are not available.

- In the hyperproliferative phase in patients with high thrombocyte counts and thromboembolic complications, cytotoxic treatment with hydroxyurea should be started.
- In the phase of bone marrow insufficiency, erythrocytes should be substituted when hemoglobin is <8 g/dL and thrombocyte transfusions should be applied when thrombocytes are $<10 \times 10^9$/L or bleeding signs appear.
- Erythropoiesis can also be stimulated with erythropoietin 3×10000 IE/week either alone or in combination with increasing doses of interferon-α three million IE subcutaneously $3\times$/week.
- Alternatively, androgens (e.g., winobanin 400–800 mg/day) can be initiated to stabilize hematopoiesis.
- Excessive splenomegaly can induce serious clinical symptoms and can be treated with irradiation or splenectomy.

Conclusions

- Standard-dose imatinib (i.e., 400 mg/day) has a comparable safety profile in elderly CML patients when compared with younger CML patients. Moreover, its clinical efficacy is also far superior to other treatment modalities, which underscores the central role of imatinib as standard first-line treatment in senior CML patients.
- Low-risk PV patients should be managed with low-dose aspirin. Special precautions should be taken in the case of patients with greater bleeding risk or allergies. Cytoreductive therapy should be considered as an option for high-risk PV patients. Hydroxyurea is the preferred agent and should be administered to maintain a platelet count of less than 600×10^9/L. If treatment with hydroxyurea is not appropriate, then either interferon or anagrelide is the option. Physicians who choose anagrelide to reduce the risk of arterial thrombosis should be aware that there are data suggesting that it is inferior to hydroxyurea, and its efficacy in comparison with no cytoreductive therapy has not been established.
- All seniors with ET are at risk for thrombotic events and should therefore be treated with hydroxyurea and low-dose aspirin. In the case hydroxyurea is not an option, anagrelide might represent an alternative treatment option, but side effects should be carefully monitored.
- Only very few senior PMF patients qualify for allogeneic stem cell transplantation, which is the only curative approach. In the hyper-proliferative phase, hydryoxyurea can reduce thrombocytosis-associated vascular events. When hematopoiesis becomes insufficient, supplementation of blood products, erythropoietin, interferon-α, or androgens can be applied to stabilize hematopoiesis.

Future Outlook

For treatment of CML, second-generation TKIs (e.g., nilotinib and dasatinib) are now available, but systematic analyses of their efficacy and safety profile in senior patients have not been performed so far. For treatment of PH-negative MPD, various JAK-2 inhibitors are currently tested in phases I to III trials, some of them showing remarkable effects in terms of spleen size reduction in patients with primary or secondary myelofibrosis. Notably, information regarding safety and clinical efficacy in elderly patients is lacking so far but should be available in future.

Declaration of Interest:

Prof Stauder has not reported any conflicts of interest.

Dr Wolf has not reported any conflicts of interest.

Further Reading

Finazzi G, Barbui T. Evidence and expertise in the management of polycythemia vera and essential thrombocythemia. Leukemia 2008; 22:1494–1502.

Gugliotta G, Castagnetti F, Amabile M, et al. Age has no impact on outcome of early chronic phase, Ph-positive CML, Imatinib treated patients: A nation-wide analysis on 559 cases of the GIMEMA CML WP. Haematologica 2009; 94 (suppl 2):256 (abstr 0632).

Harrison CN, Campbell PJ, Buck G, et al. Hydroxyurea compared with anagrelide in high-risk essential thrombocythemia. N Engl J Med 2005; 353:33–45.

Landolfi R, Marchioli R, Kutti J, et al. Efficacy and safety of low-dose aspirin in polycythemia vera. N Engl J Med 2004; 350:114–124.

Pletsch N, Lauseker M, Saussele S, et al. Therapy with Imatinib in elderly CML patients (=65 years) is well tolerated but cytogenetic and miolecular remissions seem to be achieved later compared to younger patients. Haematologica 2009; 94(suppl 2):235 (abstr 0625).

Tefferi A, Thiele J, Orazi A, et al. Proposals and rationale for revision of the World Health Organization diagnostic criteria for polycythemia vera, essential thrombocythemia, and primary myelofibrosis: recommendations from an ad hoc international expert panel. Blood 2007; 110:1092–1097.

Myelodysplastic Syndromes in the Senior Patient

11

R. Stauder and D. Wolf

Department of Internal Medicine V, Hematology and Oncology, Innsbruck Medical University, Innsbruck, Austria

The Relevance of Myelodysplastic Syndromes in the Elderly

Myelodysplastic syndromes (MDS) represent a heterogeneous group of clonal hematopoietic stem cell diseases characterized by a dysplastic and ineffective hematopoiesis. The clinical course is highly variable, ranging from mild symptoms caused by anemia, thrombocytopenia, or granulocytopenia to the transition to overt acute myeloid leukemia (AML). MDS are preferentially diagnosed in the elderly. The median age at diagnosis is 70+ in epidemiological studies (72 years in the Düsseldorf registry, 76 in the Tyrol registry, and 74 in the European Leukemia Net registry). The incidence of MDS increases dramatically with advanced age, revealing age-specific incidences of 9/100,000/yr, 25/100,000/yr, and 31/100,000/yr for the age groups 60 to 70, 71 to 80, and 80+, respectively. Moreover, therapy-related MDS (t-MDS) is observed preferentially in elderly cancer survivors following successful cytotoxic chemotherapy and/ or radiation therapy. The large and increasing proportion of elderly MDS patients and the availability of more and more treatment options impose an urgent need to develop strategies and algorithms for optimal management and treatment.

Classification and Risk Scoring in MDS

On the basis of morphologic features, MDS are classified according to the French-American-British (FAB) or World Health Organization (WHO) proposal. These classifications are based on the morphological examination of dysplastic features in hematopoietic cells, the presence of ring

Table 1 *The World Health Organization Classification of Myelodysplastic Syndromes, 2008*

Refractory cytopenias with unilineage dysplasia (RCUD)

- Refractory anemia (RA)

- Refractory neutropenia (RN)

- Refractory thrombocytopenia (RT)

Refractory anemia with ring sideroblasts (RARS; ≥15% BM ringed sideroblasts)

Refractory cytopenia with multilineage dysplasia (RCMD)

Myelodysplastic syndrome unclassified (MDS-U)

MDS associated with isolated del (5q)

Refractory anemia with excess of blasts-1 (RAEB-1, 5–9% BM blasts)

Refractory anemia with excess of blasts-2 (RAEB-2, 10–19% BM blasts)

Abbreviation: BM: bone marrow.

sideroblasts, and the percentage of bone marrow blasts. Presently, the WHO classification is most widely used (Brunning et al.) (Table 1). As the overall survival and the rate of transformation into AML vary quite considerably among patients with MDS, even within morphological subgroups, much attention has focused on the identification of additional prognostic parameters. The International Prognostic Scoring System (IPSS) has become the gold standard for clinical risk assessment in patients with primary MDS (Table 2). On the basis of the IPSS, patients are divided into low-risk (IPSS low and Int-1) and high-risk (IPSS high and Int-2) MDS. These prognostic subgroups differ significantly in survival and rates of leukemic transformation and maintain their prognostic significance even in MDS patients aged 70+. Thus, the IPSS has improved risk stratification in clinical trials and is widely used for decision-making in clinical practice. Several attempts to include additional parameters such as serum lactate dehydrogenase (LDH) or dynamic aspects like red blood cell (RBC) transfusion needs have been made to refine the IPSS. Thus, a WHO classification–based prognostic dynamic scoring system (WPSS) was described recently (Table 3). The WPSS is not only based on initial findings but also integrates evolution over time and response to

Table 2 *The Risk Score IPSS*

Prognostic variable	Score value				
	0	0,5	1	1,5	2,0
Bone marrow blasts	<5	5–10	...	11–20	21–30
Karotype[a]	Good	Intermediate	Poor		
Cytopenia[b]	0/1	2/3			

IPSS group	IPSS total score	Survival (median; yr) Age at diagnosis		25% AML evolution (yr) Age at diagnosis	
		≤70 yr	>70 yr	≤70 yr	>70 yr
Low	0	9	3,9	>9,4 (NR)	>5,8 (NR)
Intermediate-1	0,5–1,0	4,4	2,4	5,5	2,2
Intermediate-2	1,5-2	1,3	1,2	1,0	1,4
High	≥2,5	0,4	0,4	0,2	0,4

[a]Definition of karyotype:
Good   Normal, Y-, 5q-, 20q-
Intermediate   All other
Poor   Chromosome 7 aberration and/or ≥3 chromosomal aberrations
[b]Cytopenia: Hemoglobin <100 g/L (10 g/dL)
Neutrophil count <1,8 G/L (1800/µL)
Platelet count <G/L (100,000/µL)
NR, not reached
Abbreviation: IPSS, International Prognostic Scoring System.

treatment. On the basis of the total risk score, five distinct groups are defined, which are characterized by significant differences in overall survival and probability of leukemia evolution: very low-risk (score 0) (median survival 136 months), low-risk (1) (63 months), intermediate risk (2) (44 months), high risk (3,4) (19 months), and very high risk (5,6) (8 months) (Table 3).

Table 3 *The Prognostic Score WHO-based Prognostic Scoring System*

	Score value			
Variable	0	1	2	3
WHO category[a]	RA, RARS, 5q-	RCMD, RCMD-RS	RAEB-1	RAEB-2
Karyotype[b]	Good	Intermediate	Poor	-
Transfusion requirement[c]	No	Regular	-	-

[a]Based on WHO classification (Table 1)
[b]Karyotype (definition identical to International Prognostic Scoring System; Table 2)
[c]Transfussion requirement: at least one RBC transfusion every eight weeks over a period of four months
Abbreviations: WHO, World Health Organization; RBC: red blood cells.

Age-Adjusted Models and Assessment in Elderly MDS Patients

Age has a significant negative impact on overall survival in most analyses performed in MDS. In general, the relevance of age in prognostication is more pronounced in good-risk MDS than in high-risk disease. As shorter overall survival in aged persons is logical, prognostication in the elderly should include age-adjusted parameters like the standardized mortality rate (SMR) or age-adjusted survival. Thus, the survival in a given MDS patient is compared with an age- and sex-matched population. Analyses in representative cohorts of MDS patients achieved a SMR of around 5, implying a fivefold increased risk of death for MDS. Addressing various age groups, younger patients revealed an SMR of 10, and elderly an SMR of 3.4. Thus, even in elderly persons, MDS represent a relevant disease with a greater than threefold risk of disease-related death, resulting in a significant loss of life years in the majority of prognostic subgroups. However, in the prognostic excellent subgroup (WPSS very low; Table 3) of elderly patients 70+, life expectancy was not different from that in the general population, pointing out the relevance of age-matched prognostic scoring systems for designing age- and risk-adapted treatment strategies.

Whereas the scoring systems established so far are based on disease-specific prognostic factors like bone marrow blasts or karyotype, patient-related factors like functional capacities or comorbidities including cardiac insufficiency or tolerance to chemotherapy are less well defined. The integration of structured comorbidity scores to classify and quantify comorbid conditions in clinical studies has just started. The hematopoietic stem cell transplantation (HSCT)-specific comorbidity index (HCT-CI) was found to be a significant prognostic factor for overall survival as well as for event-free survival in MDS patients in uni- and in multivariate analyses and predicts nonleukemic deaths. The systematic evaluation and integration of aspects of comorbidity and functional capacities in MDS will improve individualized therapy-planning in clinical studies and in medical practice.

Treatment Options in Elderly MDS Patients

Transfusion Therapy, Growth Factors, and Iron Chelation

An essential goal in the treatment of senior MDS patients is to manage and to counteract the consequences of cytopenias and to maintain and increase the quality of life (QOL).

- Anemia is present in the vast majority (80–90%) of MDS patients and results in an impaired QOL. In addition, a high red blood cells (RBC) transfusion frequency represents an unfavorable risk factor for survival. Transfusion therapy using RBC aims to reach a range of 80 to 100 G/L in cardiorespiratory healthy persons and >100 to 120 G/L in elderly and in persons displaying comorbidities. Erythropoiesis-stimulating agents (ESAs) with or without granulocyte colony-stimulating factor (G-CSF) represent the standard of treatment for transfusion-dependent anemia in low-risk MDS (Fig. 1).

  - ESAs represent an effective treatment of anemia in MDS to improve hemoglobin levels, to reduce transfusion need, and to increase QoL. As low endogenous erythropoietin (EPO) levels as well as a low transfusion need result in an increased response rate, predictive models for ESA treatment have been developed (Table 4). The Nordic Score identifies patients with low, intermediate, and high probability of response. Moreover, G-CSF is administered in

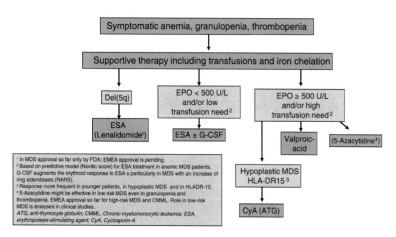

Figure I Treatment options in senior low-risk myelodysplastic syndromes (International Prognostic Scoring System low-grade and intermediate-I).

Table 4 Nordic Score to Predict Response of Erythropoiesis-Stimulating Factors in Myelodysplastic Syndromes

		Score		Score
Transfusion requirement (RBC)	<2U/months	0	≥2U/months	I
Serum Epo[a]	<500 U/L	0	≥500 U/L	I
Probability of response: Total Score 0: 74%; I: 23%; 2: 7%				

[a]Serum erythropoietin level before treatment.

combination with ESAs in low/intermediate-risk patients to augment the erythroid response, which is particularly effective in patients with an increase of ring sideroblasts (RARS). ESAs have been used safely in larger numbers of MDS patients, with no evidence for negative impact on survival or AML evolution. Moreover, ESAs even seem to improve survival in treated patients

(Jädersten et al.). When applying ESAs, the increased risk of thromboembolic complications should be considered.

- In neutropenic infections in MDS, the interventional use of G-CSF is recommended.

- In thrombopenic patients, platelet transfusions are given to prevent bleeding. However, because of immunization, frequent transfusions might cause a poor response. Thrombopoietic agents like romiplostim, which is approved for the treatment of immune thrombocytopenic purpura (ITP), have been introduced in MDS and are currently evaluated in clinical trials.

- Frequent RBC transfusions result in iron overload and may thus cause transfusion-related hemochromatosis, which primarily affects the heart and the liver. As the risk of events becomes apparent when RBC transfusions exceed 20 and serum ferritin levels exceed 1000 to 1500 ng/mL, the treatment with iron-chelating agents such as desferoxamine (applied either subcutaneously or intravenously) or deferasirox (orally) should be considered. In most guidelines, a reasonable expected survival (at least more than one year) is recommended. Renal function has to be monitored carefully in elderly patients treated with deferasirox.

Immunomodulating Agents

- Lenalidomide represents an immunomodulating drug (IMiD), which is highly active in MDS with 5q deletion. Lenalidomide produces major clinical and even cytogenetic responses, thus forming the basis for Food and Drug Agency (FDA) approval. However, actually the European Medicinal Agency (EMEA) approval is pending, as more detailed data on the safety, particularly the rate of leukemia transformation, are requested by the authorities. Lenalidomide reveals also activity in non-del5q low-risk MDS; studies to evaluate the relevance of lenalidomide in low-risk MDS are ongoing. Relevant side effects of lenalidomide are neutropenias and thrombocytopenias.

- Immunosupressive strategies using combinations of antithymocyte globulin (ATG) and cyclosporin-A (CyA) are effective in subgroups of younger patients in hypoplastic MDS and with a HLADR15 phenotype. As ATG is poorly tolerated in elderly patients, a CyA monotherapy is generally preferred. Because of nephrotoxicity, renal function has to be monitored closely.

Epigenetic Therapies

- The hypomethylating agents 5-azacytidine (AZA) and decitabine have shown encouraging results in high-risk MDS patients.
    - ¬ 5-AZA is already considered as standard of therapy in elderly high-risk MDS, who are not eligible for intensive therapies like AML induction or HSCT (Fig. 2). AZA has received an EMEA approval in MDS in this indication. In low-risk patients, these drugs are analyzed in clinical studies and might so far only be considered when signs of progression occur. AZA was demonstrated in a phase III study to significantly extend overall survival in high-risk MDS in comparison with a conventional care regimen. Effectiveness of AZA in response and survival prolongation was demonstrated in a subgroup analysis even in elderly MDS patients ($\geq$75 years). As the median number of cycles to achieve a response is three, evaluation of response should not be performed too early. In the absence of unacceptable toxicity or disease progression, continued AZA treatment might further improve responses in MDS.
- Valproic acid (VPA) was used as an anticonvulsant for decades and might be effective in myeloid neoplasms by the inhibition of histone deacetylase. As VPA causes an erythroid response in about 50% of

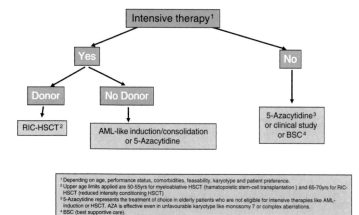

Figure 2 *Treatment options in senior high-risk myelodysplastic syndromes (International Prognostic Scoring System intermediate-2 and high-grade).*

patients in low-risk MDS, treatment with VPA might represent a useful alternative in low-risk MDS patients with a low probability of erythropoiesis-stimulating factors (ESF) response (Fig. 1). In senior patients, monitoring of VPA serum concentrations is essential.

Intensive Therapies in Elderly MDS: Current Standards

Allogeneic HSCT represents so far the only curative treatment approach in MDS. As this therapy is associated with a relatively high risk of transplant-related morbidity and mortality, a HSCT with reduced intensity conditioning (RIC-HSCT) can only be offered to a small cohort of elderly patients, who are characterized by an excellent performance status and the lack of relevant comorbidities. Similarly to HSCT, intensive AML-like polychemotherapy can restore normal polyclonal hematopoiesis in subgroups of patients but induces long-term disease-free survival only in a minority of patients. In a given elderly patient, the final decision to apply intensive therapies must be based on multiple parameters including karyotype, functional capacities, comorbidities, and patient preference (Fig. 2).

Future Perspectives

As a result of the development of innovative therapeutic options in MDS including epigenetically active drugs, immune modulating agents, thrombopoietic agents, and effective iron chelators, the treatment of elderly MDS patients has become more successful but also more complex. To choose the appropriate treatment for an elderly MDS patient, not only chronological age but also aspects of age-adjusted life expectancy, functional capacities, and comorbidities have to be integrated to achieve an individualized therapy planning and to optimize clinical outcome.

Declaration of Interest:

Dr Wolf has reported no conflicts of interest.

Further Reading

Brunning RD, Orazi A, Germing U, et al. Myelodysplastic syndromes/neoplasms overview. In: Swerdlow SH, Campo E, Harris NL, et al., eds. WHO classification of tumours of hematopoietic and lymphoid tissues. Lyon: IACR Press, 2008:88–107.

Fenaux P, Mufti GJ, Hellstrom-Lindberg E, et al. Efficacy of Azacitidine compared with that of conventional care regiment in the treatment of high risk myelodysplastic syndromes: a randomized open label phase III-study (AZA-001). International Vidaza high-risk MDS Survival Study Group. Lancet Oncol 2009; 10:223–232.

Greenberg P, Cox C, LeBeau MM, et al. International scoring system for evaluating prognosis in myelodysplastic syndromes. Blood 1997; 89:2079–2088.

Hellstrom-Lindberg E, Gulbrandsen N, Lindberg G, et al. A validated decision model for treating the anaemia of myelodysplastic syndromes with erythropoietin + granulocyte colony-stimulating factor: significant effects on quality of life. Br J Haematol 2003; 120:1037–1046.

Jädersten M, Malcovati L, Dybedal I, et al. Erythropoietin and granulocyte-colony stimulating factor treatment associated with improved survival in myelodysplastic syndrome. J Clin Oncol 2008; 26:3607–3613.

Malcovati L, Germing U, Kuendgen A, et al. Time-dependent prognostic scoring system for predicting survival and leukemic evolution in myelodysplastic syndromes. J Clin Oncol 2009; 25:3503–3510.

Nösslinger T, Tüchler H, Germing U, et al. Prognostic impact of age and gender in 897 untreated patients with primary myelodysplastic syndromes. Ann Oncol 2009; [Epub ahead of print].

Seymour JF, Fenaux P, Silverman LB, et al. Effects of Azacitidine (AZA) vs conventional care regimens (CCR) in elderly ($\geq$75 years) patients (Pts) with myelodysplastic syndromes (MDS) from the AZA-001 survival trial. Blood 2008; 112:3629.

Stauder R, Noesslinger TH, Pfeilstöcker M, et al. Impact of age and comorbidity in myelodysplastic syndromes. J Natl Compr Canc Netw 2008; 6:927–934.

Breast Cancer in the Senior Patient

12

L. Biganzoli

Medical Oncology Unit, Hospital of Prato, Istituto Tumori Toscano, Prato, Italy

Introduction

The median age for breast cancer diagnosis in Europe and in the United States is approximately 65 years. The incidence increases with increasing age.

Major limitations in defining treatment strategies in elderly breast cancer patients are the small volume of data coming from clinical trials and the heterogeneity of the older population, compounded by minimal available data for the treatment of unfit patients. There is increasing agreement that tumor biology, not chronological age, should drive treatment decisions in healthy women with breast cancer.

Early Breast Cancer

Surgery

The surgical approach in older patients with breast cancer should not differ from that in younger women. Depending on the clinical situation, breast-conserving surgery or mastectomy combined with sentinel node biopsy or axillary dissection are proper options. It is worth mentioning that a very low local recurrence rate has been observed in patients with clinically node-negative, hormone receptor–positive, early breast cancer who received tamoxifen and no axillary clearance. This approach remains exploratory and should be reserved for patients who present contraindications to or refuse a standard approach.

Primary Endocrine Therapy

Primary hormonal therapy can be considered only in really frail patients with endocrine-sensitive tumors since this approach has been shown to be inferior to surgery in fit women.

Radiotherapy

There is no evidence of increased toxicity related to the use of radiotherapy in elderly patients. Radiotherapy should be considered after conservative surgery and postmastectomy for T3-T4 tumors or involvement of four or more axillary lymph nodes. The benefit of radiation therapy over tamoxifen alone is limited mainly to a decrease in local relapse. This decrease is also significant, even if small (3% in 5 years), in patients older than 70 years with receptor-positive, pT1N0 invasive breast cancer and clear margins. The cost:benefit ratio of postmastectomy radiotherapy should be discussed in patients with limited life expectancy (less than five years).

Adjuvant Endocrine Treatment

Endocrine therapy is effective in elderly patients with hormone receptor–positive tumors. The benefit of tamoxifen is age independent. Similarly, there is no differential effect of age on the efficacy and safety of aromatase inhibitors. Tumor biology, risk of relapse, and comorbidities should be considered in selecting the preferred approach, consisting of single-agent tamoxifen, that is, low-risk tumor and osteoporosis, upfront aromatase inhibitor, or a sequential strategy. The extended approach, namely administration of an aromatase inhibitor after five years of treatment with tamoxifen, is associated with a significant advantage in terms of disease-free survival only in patients younger than 60 years (trial MA.17). However, the study showed no interaction between treatment and age, indicating a probable similar effect of the aromatase inhibitor among all age groups.

Older patients with low-risk breast cancer, specifically T < 1 cm, N0, or who have a limited life expectancy, that is, less than 10 years, are unlikely to derive any survival benefit from endocrine therapy.

Adjuvant Chemotherapy

The benefit of adjuvant chemotherapy progressively decreases with increasing age. The benefit experienced by patients aged 70 years and older is in the same range as those aged 50 to 70 years.

- In general, patients with hormone receptor–negative tumors benefit more from chemotherapy than patients with hormone receptor–positive tumors. Two retrospective studies, based on data from the Surveillance, Epidemiology, and End Results (SEER) database, have shown an advantage in terms of overall survival from adjuvant chemotherapy in elderly patients with estrogen-receptor negative tumors. In one of the two studies, the benefit was observed only in patients with node-positive tumors.

- As in the younger population, the additive value of chemotherapy to endocrine therapy is possibly confined to tumors that are not completely endocrine sensitive.
- In the National Surgical Adjuvant Breast and Bowel Project (NSABP) B-20, no additional benefit was gained from adjuvant chemotherapy in older patients. Subsequent application of a genetic signature (OncotypeDx) suggested that this lack of benefit was due not to age but to a higher proportion of older patients with a more favorable profile for endocrine responsiveness.

Regarding the choice of chemotherapy regimen, a recent randomized clinical trial conducted in breast cancer patients aged 65 years and older has shown that, as in younger women, polychemotherapy [doxorubin and cyclophosphamide (AC) × 4 cycles; or classical cyclophosphamide, methotrexate, and fluorouracil (CMF) × 6 cycles] is superior to single-agent adjuvant chemotherapy (capecitabine).

Also, it should be mentioned that in comparison with less intensive poly-chemotherapy regimens, intensive regimens in patients aged 65 years and older (CMF plus vincristine and prednisone; high-dose cyclophosphamide with doxorubicin and fluorouracil; or AC followed by paclitaxel) are associated with a reduced therapeutic index (same efficacy but increased treatment-related mortality). Adjuvant docetaxel and cyclophosphamide (TC) is superior to AC also in older patients (≥65 years). Febrile neutropenia has been reported in 8% of elderly patients treated with TC.

Tumor biology, risk of relapse, and patient's life expectancy, rather than age, must influence clinical decision-making and determine the appropriateness of adjuvant chemotherapy for an elderly woman with breast cancer. Healthy older patients with node-positive, hormone receptor–negative tumors derive the largest benefit from adjuvant chemotherapy. There is no evidence of benefit from adjuvant chemotherapy in unfit patients.

Trastuzumab

Few patients aged 70 years or over have been included in trials evaluating the role of trastuzumab in the adjuvant setting. The recommendations of the International Society of Geriatric Oncology (SIOG) are to offer, in the absence of cardiac contraindications, adjuvant trastuzumab to older patients with HER2-positive breast cancer when chemotherapy is indicated. Cardiac monitoring is considered essential. No data support the use of adjuvant trastuzumab with endocrine therapy without chemotherapy.

Locally Advanced Breast Cancer

The approach in healthy older patients with locally advanced breast cancer should not differ from that in younger women. The choice of the chemotherapy regimen is influenced by an individual patient's characteristics. Regarding the use of trastuzumab, the same approach outlined in the adjuvant setting is applicable. In the case of neoadjuvant endocrine therapy, an aromatase inhibitor is the agent of choice.

Metastatic Breast Cancer

Endocrine Therapy

Endocrine therapy is the treatment of choice for women with hormone receptor–positive, non-life-threatening disease. In patients with response or prolonged disease stabilization from hormonal therapy, the use of a subsequent line of non-cross-resistant endocrine therapy is considered an adequate strategy at the time of disease progression. Several treatment options are available: tamoxifen, an aromatase inhibitor (including a switch from a nonsteroidal to a steroidal aromatase inhibitor in the setting of progression), fulvestrant, progestins, and androgens.

Chemotherapy

Chemotherapy is the treatment of choice in patients with hormone receptor–negative, endocrine-resistant, or rapidly proliferating disease.

- Polychemotherapy is recommended in patients in whom rapid tumor reduction is needed.
- Single-agent chemotherapy is preferable in asymptomatic patients with a low tumor burden or in unfit patients.

Cytotoxic agents with a favorable safety profile, for example, weekly taxanes or anthracyclines, liposomal doxorubicin, capecitabine, vinorelbine, or gemcitabine are recommended. Personalized treatments, specifically dose reductions to improve the therapeutic index of treatments, can be considered in unfit patients. Elderly patients present decreased tolerance to treatment. Close monitoring of toxicity is recommended.

Biological Agents

- In the absence of cardiac contraindication, trastuzumab can be safely administered to elderly patients with HER2+, metastatic breast cancer.
  - ¬ In fit patients, concurrent administration of trastuzumab and chemotherapy is recommended.
  - ¬ Trastuzumab plus an aromatase inhibitor represents an interesting option for patients with HER2+, hormone receptor–positive, indolent disease or for patients considered unfit for chemotherapy.
  - ¬ Single-agent trastuzumab may be considered in women with HER2+, hormone receptor–negative disease who are not considered candidates for or who refuse chemotherapy.
- Because of limited data on the combination of capecitabine plus lapatinib in older patients, this association should be considered only in women with good performance status. Extremely interesting are the preliminary data presented on the combination of lapatinib and letrozole.
- The addition of bevacizumab to first-line chemotherapy improves progression-free survival in advanced breast cancer. Age-based subanalyses have been conducted in three clinical trials evaluating bevacizumab in combination with chemotherapy, mainly taxanes. Comparable efficacy between younger and older patients was observed in two studies, while the effect of bevacizumab declined with age in a trial evaluating the antiangiogenic agent in combination with weekly paclitaxel. The safety profile of bevacizumab in older patients has been extensively evaluated in an observational study with reassuring results. A slight increase in the incidence of hypertension was reported in patients aged 70 years and older in comparison with younger patients. Of note, approximately 50% of the older patients entered in this trial had preexisting hypertension documented at study commencement.

Bisphosphonates

The use of bisphosphonates in patients with metastatic bone lesions is indicated irrespective of age.

Conclusions

There is increasing evidence that a selected population of elderly breast cancer patients may benefit from specific anticancer therapies both in the adjuvant and metastatic settings. Data do not support the use of adjuvant chemotherapy or trastuzumab in unfit patients. Questionable is the benefit of adjuvant endocrine therapy in unfit patients or older patients at very low risk of relapse. A personalized approach that takes into account both the tumor and the patient's characteristics (e.g., tumor burden, presence of symptoms), as well as patient's preferences, should be considered in unfit patients with advanced disease.

Declaration of Interest:

Dr Biganzoli has reported no conflicts of interest.

Further Reading

Crivellari D, Aapro M, Leonard R, et al. Breast cancer in the elderly: Making the right decision. J Clin Oncol 2007; 25:1882–1890.

Early Breast Cancer Trialists' Collaborative Group. Effects of chemotherapy and hormonal therapy for early breast cancer on recurrence and 15-year survival: an overview of the randomised trials. Lancet 2005; 365:1687–1717.

Jones S, Holmes FA, O'Shaughnessy J, et al. Docetaxel with cyclophosphamide is associated with an overall survival benefit compared with doxorubicin and cyclophosphamide: 7-year follow-up of US Oncology Research Trial 9735. J Clin Oncol 2009; 27(8):1177–1183.

Muss HB, Berry DA, Cirrincione CT, et al. Adjuvant chemotherapy in older women with early-stage breast cancer. N Engl J Med 2009; 360:2055–2065.

Muss H, Biganzoli L, Sargent D, et al. Adjuvant therapy in the elderly: making the right decision. J Clin Oncol 2007; 25:1870–1875.

Wildiers H, Kunkler I, Biganzoli L, et al. Management of breast cancer in elderly individuals: recommendations of the International Society of Geriatric Oncology. Lancet Oncol 2007; 8:1101–1115.

Lung Cancer in the Elderly

D. Schrijvers

Department of Hemato-Oncology, Ziekenhuisnetwerk
Antwerpen-Middelheim, Antwerp, Belgium

Introduction

Lung cancer is the most common cancer in the world, and the majority of lung cancer patients are above the age of 65 years. The changing demographics will result in an even higher number of senior people who will develop lung cancer and are in need of subsequent cancer treatment and care. This patient population may suffer from other comorbid conditions or geriatric syndromes, complicating their treatment and care.

While there are some data from randomized trials including fit senior patients, there is only a limited amount of information regarding vulnerable or frail elderly.

Early Non–Small Cell Lung Cancer in the Elderly

Without treatment, the five-year overall survival rate in patients with stage I non–small cell cancer (NSCLC) is between 6% and 14% with a five-year disease-specific survival rate of 23% for T1 tumors. Anticancer treatment can improve these figures but should be used carefully in the elderly.

Lung Cancer Surgery

Retrospective studies show that age alone should not be an exclusion criterion for surgery.

- In 10,761 patients with stage IA NSCLC tumor size, gender, age, and extent of resection were significant predictors of survival in uni- and multivariate analysis: patients older than 67 years had a worse five-year survival than those under 67 years (52% vs. 65%; $p < 0.0001$)

- In 19,702 patients with stage IA and IB NSCLC, advanced age at diagnosis, male sex, low socioeconomic status, nonsurgical treatment, and poor histological grade [stage IA NSCLC: hazard ratio (HR) 1.13, 95% confidence interval (CI) 1.08–1.19; stage IB NSCLC: HR 1.11; 95% CI 1.07–1.16] were associated with an increased risk of mortality on multivariate analysis.
- The age-related mortality and the long-term survival in 2,021 patients who underwent major pulmonary resections (lobectomy, pneumonectomy) as treatment with curative intent for primary NSCLC were not significantly influenced by age when three age categories (<65 years, 65–75, and >75 years) were compared. There was a slight increase in mortality with increasing age.
  - ˥ After lobectomy mortality was 0.9% in patients aged <65 years, 1.9% in patients aged 65 to 75 years, and 4.0% in patients aged >75 years.
  - ˥ After pneumonectomy these figures were 3.0%, 7.9%, and 10.5%, respectively.

  The overall five-year survival rates were 52.5%, 45.8%, and 50% for the respective groups, with no significant difference among them. An impaired performance status (ECOG status grades 1–3) had a significant negative impact on survival in subjects older than 65 years ($p = 0.017$) and in subjects older than 75 years ($p = 0.002$).
- Other factors predicting a negative outcome of surgery are a Karnofsky performance score <70%, a forced expiratory volume in the first second (FEV_1) <60% of the predicted value or FEV_1 <1 L, arterial blood gas Pao_2 <60 mmHg, and $Paco_2$ >40 mmHg.

After adequate selection, senior patients can undergo lung cancer surgery, although a slight increase in mortality should be anticipated.

Radiotherapy

Radiotherapy is a valid treatment option in patients unfit for or unwilling to undergo surgery.

- Conventional radiotherapy results in local recurrence rates as high as 40% (range 6–70%), and three-year overall and cause-specific survival rates of 34% and 39%, respectively.

- Stereotactic radiotherapy results in a local control rate of 90% and a five-year overall survival rate of 70.8%. Acute toxicities are mild with fatigue, nausea, and chest pain; late toxicities exceeding grade II (National Cancer Institute Common Toxicity Criteria version 3) are limited to <10% of patients and are mainly observed with large or centrally located tumors. Radiation pneumonitis exceeding grade 2 develops in 3% of patients, while rib fractures and chronic pain syndromes located at the chest wall are also described.

Radiotherapy should be proposed to patients with local disease who are not candidates for surgery.

Adjuvant Chemotherapy

Several large phase III randomized trials and meta-analysis have established the role of adjuvant cisplatin-based combination chemotherapy in early-stage NSCLC with an improvement of 5.3% in five-year survival in patients with stages II to IIIA disease. However, there are no data of prospective, elderly-specific trials.

- In the randomized trials, age seemed not to be an important factor influencing disease-free and overall survival: subgroup analysis of the meta-analysis showed that the benefit of adjuvant chemotherapy was independent of age and that elderly (up to age 75 years) derived similar benefits from adjuvant chemotherapy as younger patients.
- The retrospective analysis of the study JBR.10 by the National Cancer Institute of Canada (NCIC) Clinical Trials Group showed that, despite the fact that elderly patients were receiving less chemotherapy, adjuvant vinorelbine and cisplatin also improved five-year survival in patients older than 65 years (68% vs. 48%; HR death 0.61; $p = 0.04$) with acceptable toxicity. Patients aged more than 75 years had significantly shorter survival than those aged 66 to 74 years (HR death 1.95; $p = 0.02$).
- In another trial, the benefit of adjuvant chemotherapy was not seen in the age group >65 years.

In selected elderly patients, adjuvant chemotherapy might be of benefit, although there is a need for elderly-specific, prospective trials.

Chemoradiation

Several randomized trials have compared sequential and concurrent chemoradiation with radiotherapy alone and demonstrated the superiority of combined-modality approaches. Recent randomized trials have also compared sequential with concurrent approaches, demonstrating a survival benefit in favor of concurrent chemoradiation.

Relatively limited elderly-specific prospective data are available, but several phase II studies have shown that alternative schedules and doses may be used in elderly patients, and low-dose chemotherapy as well as noncisplatin regimens are active and feasible in the elderly.

Retrospective analyses of randomized trials of chemoradiation have compared treatment outcomes between elderly patients and younger patients. Results are inconsistent, with some analyses showing an excess of toxicity and a lack of survival benefit in the elderly, while others confirm both the feasibility and efficacy of combined-modality treatment in this population, including the more toxic concurrent schedules, and still others demonstrating increased toxicity but survival rates equivalent to younger individuals.

Advanced Non–Small Cell Lung Cancer in the Elderly

When choosing a treatment strategy in elderly patients with advanced NSCLC, several options are available such as palliative care without chemotherapy, single-agent chemotherapy with a third-generation drug, non-platinum-based combination chemotherapy, platinum-based combination chemotherapy, and new biologic agents.

Single-Agent Chemotherapy

Single-agent chemotherapy with vinorelbine, gemcitabine, and taxanes (paclitaxel and docetaxel) are first-line treatment options supported by prospective, elderly-specific clinical data (Table 1).

Combination Chemotherapy

To improve the results obtained with single-agent chemotherapy in elderly patients, several strategies have been tested: sequential single-agent treatment or combination therapy.

Table 1 *Randomized Trials in Elderly Patients with Advanced Non-Small Cell Lung Cancer*

Author (yr)	Treatment	Number of patients	Response rate (%)	Median overall survival (wk)	Quality of life/ toxicity
First-line treatment					
Elvis (99)	Best supportive care	78		21	⇑ Vinorelbine
	Vinorelbine	76	20	28	
Frasci (00)	Vinorelbine	60	15	18	⇑ Vinorelbine + gemcitabine
	Vinorelbine + gemcitabine	60	22	29	
Gridelli (03)	Vinorelbine	223	18	36	=
	Gemcitabine	223	16	28	
	Vinorelbine + gemcitabine	232	21	30	
Kudoh (06)	Vinorelbine	91	10	57	⇑ Docetaxel
	Docetaxel	91	23	39	
Chen (06)	Carbo + paclitaxel	40	40	41	Cisplatin more toxic than carboplatin
	Cis + paclitaxel	41	39	42	

Study	Treatment	N			Comments
Hainsworth (07)	Docetaxel	345		20	=
	Docetaxel + gemcitabine			22	
Leong (07)	Gemcitabine	43	16		=
	Vinorelbine	45	20		
	Docetaxel	46	22		
Gridelli (07)	Pemetrexed	44	4.5	18	=
	Pemetrexed + gemcitabine	43	11.6	23	
Lilenbaum (07)	Docetaxel q 1 wk × 3 q28 days	56		14	3-weekly more toxic than 1-weekly
	Docetaxel q 3 wk	55		25	
Ramalingam (08)	Carbo + paclitaxel	113	17	49	⇓ Bevacizumab
	Carbo + paclitaxel + bevacizumab	111	29	45	
Second- or third-line treatment					
Wheatley (08)	Erlotinib	112	7.6	31	⇑ Erlotinib
	Placebo	51	NA	20	

Abbreviations: ⇑, better for; q, every; ⇓, worse for; wk, week; carbo, carboplatin; cis, cisplatin; NA, not available; =, equal; d, day.

Sequential Chemotherapy

In a phase II study, elderly patients aged ≥ 70 years were treated with three cycles of gemcitabine [1200 mg/m^2 d1, d8 every (q) three weeks] followed by three cycles of docetaxel (37 mg/m^2 d1, d8 q three weeks). The objective response rate was 16.0% (95%CI 7.6–28.3%), with a median time to progression of 4.8 months (95%CI 3.6–6.0 months) and median duration of survival of 8.0 months (95%CI 5.6–10.5 months). No grade 4 hematological toxicity was observed, and grade 3 neutropenia and thrombocytopenia were reported in 5.4% and 3.6% of the patients, respectively. Sequential gemcitabine and docetaxel seem a well-tolerated and effective regimen.

The sequential administration of pemetrexed followed by gemcitabine was compared with pemetrexed alone in elderly or patients younger than 70 years but ineligible for platinum-based chemotherapy. Patients were treated in the sequential arm with pemetrexed for cycles 1 and 2 and then with gemcitabine (1200 mg/m^2 d1, d8 q three weeks) for cycles 3 and 4 (repeated once for a total of eight cycles). The tumor response rate was 11.6%, the median progression-free survival time 3.3 months, and the median overall survival time 5.4 months with a one-year survival rate of 28.1%. Grade 3/4 hematologic toxicity consisted of neutropenia (2.3%), febrile neutropenia (4.7%), thrombocytopenia (7.0%), and anemia (4.7%). There was no difference with single-agent pemetrexed.

Non-Platinum-Based Combinations

Several non-platinum-based combinations have been developed in phase II studies combining gemcitabine with vinorelbine, docetaxel, or paclitaxel in different treatment schedules.

When these combinations were compared with single-agent treatment, the combination arm resulted, sometimes, in higher response rates or disease-free survival but not in higher median overall survival or one-year survival rates (Table 1). Combination treatment was also slightly more toxic than single-agent treatment.

Platinum-Based Combinations

- Cisplatin-based chemotherapy is currently recommended as the standard treatment for patients with advanced NSCLC. However, no prospective phase III study has shown a benefit in elderly patients. Cisplatin administration is associated with significant hematologic and nonhematologic toxicity (e.g., nephrotoxicity, ototoxicity, and neurotoxicity).

- Carboplatin has a lower rate of emesis, nephrotoxicity, and neurotoxicity but causes more hematologic toxicity, particularly if combined with other myelotoxic agents.

Several platinum combinations have been tested in elderly patients, but only a limited number of prospective randomized clinical trials of platinum-based chemotherapy with inclusion criteria limited to the elderly population have been performed (Table 1). These show that platinum-based combinations are feasible in selected elderly patients.

Targeted Therapy

Targeted therapies are an alternative to chemotherapy in the treatment of elderly advanced NSCLC patients because of the safety profile of most of these new drugs. However, medication interfering with the vascular endothelial growth factor receptor pathway can induce hypertension and bleeding and should be used with caution in elderly patients.

- Erlotinib, an epidermal growth factor receptor inhibitor, was tested in a phase II study in 80 patients older than 70 years of age with previously untreated advanced NSCLC. It was well tolerated and demonstrated a response rate of 10% and a disease stabilization rate of 41%. There was a significant improvement of symptoms (dyspnea, cough, fatigue, and pain) and a median survival time of 10.9 months. Rash and diarrhea were the most common toxicities, occurring in 81% and 69% of the patients, respectively.
- Bevacizumab in combination with carboplatin and paclitaxel was compared with carboplatin and paclitaxel in patients 70 years and older with advanced NSCLC. There were no differences in response rate or median overall survival, but grade 3 to 5 toxicities occurred in 87% of elderly patients with bevacizumab versus 61% with carboplatin and paclitaxel alone ($p < 0.001$), with seven treatment-related deaths in the bevacizumab arm compared with two in the control arm. Patients had higher incidence of grade 3 to 5 neutropenia, bleeding, and proteinuria with bevacizumab compared with younger patients.

Second- and Third-Line Treatment

Second-line therapy seems to be possible in elderly patients, as shown by a retrospective analysis of a phase III trial of pemetrexed versus docetaxel in the second-line treatment of advanced NSCLC showing a similar outcome in elderly and younger patients.

In a subgroup analysis of second- or third-line erlotinib after chemotherapy, there was no difference among age groups, and patients older than 70 years had the same benefit as younger patients. Elderly patients, compared with young patients, had significantly more overall and severe (grade 3 and 4) toxicity (35% vs. 18%; $p < 0.001$), were more likely to discontinue treatment as a result of treatment-related toxicity (12% vs. 3%; $p < 0.0001$), and had lower relative dose intensity (64% vs. 82% received >90% planned dose; $p < 0.001$).

Small Cell Lung Cancer in the Elderly

The standard therapy for limited-disease (LD) small cell lung cancer (SCLC) is four to six cycles of a platinum-based chemotherapy regimen combined with concurrent thoracic radiotherapy of the tumor region and the mediastinum. Chemotherapy remains the only treatment for patients affected by extensive-disease (ED) SCLC.

After response, prophylactic cranial irradiation results in a survival benefit in both LD and ED SCLC.

In elderly the standard cisplatin-based regimens lead to substantial toxicity, and these regimens are only indicated in the very fit senior patients. Many authors found that older patients (70 years) treated with optimal chemotherapy had response rates and overall survival rates similar to those in younger patients, although the elderly received less chemotherapy than the planned protocol and experienced more toxicity.

The addition of radiotherapy to chemotherapy should be carefully considered: a meta-analysis showed that thoracic radiotherapy moderately improved survival (5.4% ± 1.4% at three years), but this effect was lost in patients ≥70 years of age.

Alternative treatments in elderly patients are single-agent treatments or non-cisplatin-containing combinations.

- Single-agent activity has been reported with oral etoposide (response rate 53–84%; median survival time 4.6–16 months), epirubicin (response rate 45–55%; median survival time 6 months), and carboplatin (response rate 25.4%; median survival time 3.9 months). These single-agent treatments had a worse treatment outcome when compared with combination therapy.
- Several phase II trials were performed in elderly patients, with the combination of carboplatin plus etoposide being the most investigated. They showed a good activity, with response rates ranging from 59% to 81% and a median survival time ranging from 7.9 to 11.6 months but substantial myelotoxicity. When compared with cisplatin (25 mg/m^2 d1–3) plus etoposide (80 mg/m^2 d1–3), the carboplatin (AUC5) combination had a similar response rate (73/73%) and median overall survival (10.6/9.9 months; $p = 0.54$). Toxicity was manageable with the use of hematologic growth factors.
- Several phase II trials have been performed with third-generation combination chemotherapy and specific regimens for the elderly with varying success.

Palliative Treatment in Elderly Lung Cancer Patients

Palliative radiotherapy is commonly employed in the treatment of lung cancer. This is particularly true for older patients who may not be suitable for definitive or curative treatment approaches. Several symptoms including hemoptysis, dyspnea, and cough and chest pain are best palliated by short-course radiotherapy. This also prevents disease progression with lung collapse or other consequences. Poor prognostic factors such as performance status, age, or stage have little impact on achieving palliation. Therefore, palliative treatment should be offered to all, irrespective of poor prognostic factors since the benefits of palliative radiotherapy are similar in the elderly compared with younger patients.

All patients with incurable lung cancer should receive palliative care for symptom control.

Conclusion

Senior patients with lung cancer should receive optimal anticancer treatment. When fit, most of them will support standard treatment with some modification or extra supportive care. Data on anticancer treatment in the elderly lung cancer population are increasingly available, and treatment decisions can be made on evidence-based data.

However, for vulnerable and frail elderly, treatment strategies should be developed and adapted to these patients to ensure an optimal treatment and care and improvement of their quality of life.

Declaration of Interest:
Dr Schrijvers has not reported any conflicts of interest.

Further Reading

Gridelli C, Langer C, Maione P, et al. Lung cancer in the elderly. J Clin Oncol 2007; 25:1898–1907.

Langer CJ. Resectable non-small cell lung cancer in the elderly: is there a role for adjuvant treatment? Drugs Aging 2008; 25:209–218.

Muss HB, Biganzoli L, Sargent DJ, et al. Adjuvant therapy in the elderly: making the right decision. J Clin Oncol 2007; 25:1870–1875.

Rossi A, Maione P, Colantuoni G, et al. Treatment of small cell lung cancer in the elderly. Oncologist 2005; 10:399–411.

Schild SE, Stella PJ, Geyer SM, et al. The outcome of combined-modality therapy for stage III non-small-cell lung cancer in the elderly. J Clin Oncol 2003; 21:3201–3206.

Turner NJ, Muers MF, Haward RA, et al. Do elderly people with lung cancer benefit from palliative radiotherapy? Lung Cancer 2005; 49:193–202.

Owonikoko TK, Ramalingam S. Small cell lung cancer in elderly patients: a review. J Natl Compr Canc Netw 2008; 6:333–344.

Colorectal Cancer

D. Papamichael
Department of Medical Oncology, B.O. Cyprus Oncology Centre, Nicosia, Cyprus

Introduction

Cancer incidence is expected to increase dramatically in the 21st century. The increase is likely to be driven largely by cancers diagnosed in senior adults. This is particularly true for colorectal cancer (CRC), where approximately 50% of cases are diagnosed in patients older than 70 years of age, with a median age at diagnosis of about 71 years. The relative survival of senior CRC patients is worse than that of younger individuals, possibly because of a more advanced stage at presentation but quite often suboptimal management. Concerns over existing comorbidities, physical or mental frailty, and age-specific deteriorating organ function are often cited as reasons for senior CRC patients not receiving "optimal" treatment. Indeed, senior CRC patients have so far been underrepresented in clinical trials, and therefore, extrapolation of such results to this group of patients can only be made with caution. The data for patients over the age of 75 years appear especially sparse. The difficulties and potential pitfalls in managing senior CRC patients in the adjuvant and advanced disease setting will be considered.

Adjuvant Chemotherapy

A substantial proportion of patients with stage I or II CRC can be cured by surgery alone, although a small number of patients with stage II disease can derive additional benefit from adjuvant chemotherapy.

On the other hand, the administration of adjuvant chemotherapy to patients with node-positive colon cancer has clearly been shown to significantly improve disease-free and overall survival. Nevertheless, the use of such treatment in patients over 70 years of age remains controversial because of concerns over both toxicity and death from causes unrelated to cancer.

- Retrospective data collected from the Surveillance, Epidemiology, and End Results (SEER) registry and Medicare database in the United States, which included very large numbers of individuals, suggest that patients over the age of 65 to 70 derived a similar benefit to their younger counterparts, even though they were less likely to receive treatment and were more likely to discontinue their treatment before the "standard-of-care" six months.
- Data from Europe, on the other hand, suggest that quality of life is not likely to be affected more adversely in senior CRC patients receiving adjuvant therapy.
- In a pooled analysis from seven studies of the North Surgical Adjuvant Breast and Bowel Project (NSABP) where 3,351 patients received 5-fluorouracil (5FU)-based chemotherapy, no significant interaction was observed between age and efficacy of treatment, and the incidence of toxicity was not increased in patients over 70 years, except for leucopenia in one study. However, an analysis on the probability of death without cancer in the same study was shown to be strongly associated with age, with patients over 70 having a 13% chance of dying from other causes without recurrent disease.
- The randomized X-ACT trial of bolus 5FU plus leucovorin (LV) versus capecitabine in patients with stage III disease and with an upper age limit of 75 years showed no difference in terms of safety for patients over and under 65 years. A recent update of the same study identified age as a non-significant factor for overall survival in a multivariate analysis.
- In addition, another retrospective review from a single institution suggested that patients over 70 years were more likely to experience mucositis when bolus 5FU was used.
- In the MOSAIC trial of adjuvant oxaliplatin/5FU/LV (FOLFOX) versus FU/LV, age had no impact on the relative benefit of FOLFOX on recurrence-free survival. Senior CRC patients had the same benefit from treatment as their younger counterparts, although the eligibility was limited to 75 years, and all patients were deemed fit to enter a clinical trial. More recently, a pooled analysis of the ACCENT database was presented in abstract form, using data from 10,499 patients <70 years

and 2170 patients >70 years participating in six phase III adjuvant trials comparing intravenous 5FU/LV with combinations of irinotecan, oxaliplatin, or oral 5FU analogues in stages II and III colon cancer. All outcome measures (including disease-free and overall survival) were statistically significantly improved for the younger patients in the experimental arms but not for senior CRC patients, with the interaction between age and treatment being statistically significant for all endpoints. The authors concluded that senior patients do not receive the same benefit from combination treatments or oral fluoropyrimidines as their younger counterparts. Nevertheless, the above results should be interpreted with caution, as no information was provided on disease-specific survival, toxicity and dose-intensity in this analysis. Any potential survival gain in the senior patient population can be difficult to ascertain because of an increase in deaths from other causes.

- The situation in patients with stage II disease is even less clear with respect to senior CRC patients and the potential impact of adjuvant therapy. A recent publication from the QUASAR Collaborative Group suggests that the net benefit from adjuvant chemotherapy in this group is likely to be extremely small even with the highest estimate for treatment efficacy.

Therefore, it is difficult to recommend adjuvant therapy for all senior CRC patients. The evidence so far for senior CRC patients' ability to tolerate chemotherapy in general suggests that age alone should not exclude any stage III colon cancer patient from the consideration of adjuvant therapy. On the other hand, for patients over 75 for whom there are very little data so far, age alone may well be a legitimate consideration. In any case, the therapeutic decisions with regard to whether to treat or not and choice of adjuvant therapy should be reached jointly by patient and physician taking into account individual preferences and existing comorbidities.

Metastatic Disease

The treatment of advanced CRC has seen a rapid succession of significant advances over the last few years. The introduction of novel conventional cytotoxic agents such is oxaliplatin and irinotecan and, more recently, the antiangiogenic agent bevacizumab and two epidermal growth factor receptor antibodies, namely cetuximab and panitumumab, comprise a rapidly changing treatment landscape. However, as a consequence of the underrepresentation of senior CRC patients in clinical trials, our knowledge of the performance of the appropriate therapeutic strategies in this age group is often very limited.

- Retrospective data have shown that older and younger patients with metastatic CRC derive similar benefit from 5FU-based chemotherapy. The same data have suggested better efficacy for infusional 5FU as opposed to the bolus regimens.
- More recent data concerning the addition of irinotecan to 5FU for patients over and under 70 years showed toxicity and efficacy to be broadly similar in the two age groups. A pooled analysis for the use of FOLFOX in the context of randomized trials in senior (>70 years) as compared with younger (<70 years) metastatic CRC patients showed the combination regimen to maintain its efficacy and safety ratio in most patients over 70 years. Generally, it appears that with careful monitoring for toxicity and rapid intervention, there is probably no reason why senior CRC patients should not receive either irinotecan- or oxaliplatin-based treatment unless other contraindications for chemotherapy exist.
- More recently, studies have been specifically designed for senior CRC patients to assess the role of single-agent versus combination chemotherapy in the metastatic setting. Hopefully, these will provide additional useful information on patterns of toxicity and efficacy in the metastatic setting.
- Relatively limited data from studies of the three targeted agents currently approved for use in the treatment of metastatic CRC, namely bevacizumab, cetuximab, and panitumumab, suggest that they are probably safe in a senior patient population. However, arterial thromboembolic events with the use of bevacizumab are more likely to occur in those aged over 65 years of age or those who have a previous history of such events (>18%). In these categories, it may be considered appropriate to omit the antiangiogenic agent and go for a different treatment strategy.

Liver resection offers the only chance for long-term survival or even cure for patients with metastases confined to the liver. Retrospective data from the LiverMetSurvey registry and other single institution data suggest that well-selected senior CRC patients stand to gain almost equally from liver metastasectomy as their younger counterparts, even though perioperative mortality may be somewhat worse. The use of perioperative chemotherapy in potentially resectable liver disease is currently gaining significant ground, although no senior CRC patients have been included in any of the recent trials and there are potential tolerance issues with the more active triple regimens or chemotherapy combinations plus biologics.

Conclusion

Overall, cytotoxic chemotherapy should not be denied to senior CRC patients with either early or advanced disease. It should be noted, however, that much of the data currently available are based on age-specific retrospective analyses and are likely to suffer from selection bias. Results from clinical trials conducted in younger patients cannot be extrapolated to the general senior patient population. Ideally, prospective, senior-specific clinical trials should be designed and conducted to provide evidence-based recommendations for the management of this specific patient population.

Declaration of Interest:

Dr Papamichael has reported no conflicts of interest.

Further Reading

Köhne CH, Folprecht G, Goldberg R, et al. Chemotherapy in elderly patients with colorectal cancer. Oncologist 2008; 13:390–402.
Papamichael D, Audisio R, Horiot JC, et al. Treatment of the elderly colorectal cancer patient: SIOG expert recommendations. Ann Oncol 2009; 20:5–16.
Sanoff H, Bleiberg H, Goldberg R, et al. Managing older patients with colorectal cancer. J Clin Oncol 2007; 25:1891–1897.

Prostate Cancer

C. Terret
PROLOG (Pilot Unit of Oncogeriatry in Lyon), Department of Medical Oncology, Université de Lyon, Centre Léon Bérard, Lyon, France

A. Fléchon
Urologic Oncology Program, Department of Medical Oncology, Université de Lyon, Centre Léon Bérard, Lyon, France

J.P. Droz
Department of Medical Oncology, Université de Lyon, Centre Léon Bérard, Lyon, France

Introduction and General Background

Prostate cancer is predominantly a disease of senior adults (i.e., men aged 70 years or older), yet, no specific guidelines exist for this population.

Existing guidelines for the management of prostate cancer make little reference to senior adult patients and age-related factors that may affect treatment decisions. Some, like the European Association of Urology (EAU) guidelines, refer to the concept of life expectancy, which depends on many components of a patient's well-being and is often misinterpreted by physicians. Nevertheless, guidelines for assessing the health status of senior adults have been published and can be applied to patients with prostate cancer.

Epidemiology

Prostate cancer is the most frequently diagnosed male cancer in Europe and represents the third cause of cancer-related death in men. The median age at diagnosis is 68 years; over 60% of new cases are diagnosed in men ≥65 years of age and 25.7% in men ≥75 years of age.

The overall growth and "aging" of the world's population are expected to increase the burden of prostate cancer—particularly in senior adults. In more developed regions of the world, the proportion of men aged ≥70 years is expected to increase from 0.8% in the year 2000 to 17.2% by 2050.

Diagnosis and Staging

The diagnosis of prostate cancer is often made at the occasion of an individual screening examination. Otherwise, it is made when urological symptoms occur or when metastatic disease to bone becomes painful. The diagnosis is made on prostate biopsy. Extension evaluation is based on prognostic factor study and sometimes on abdominal and pelvis computed tomography (CT) scan, prostate magnetic resonance imaging (MRI), and bone scan.

Prognosis

Prognostic factors of localized prostate cancer are clinical TNM stage, initial serum prostate-specific antigen (PSA) value, and tumor grade (Gleason score). This evaluation allows to classify the patients in prognostic groups, as described by D'Amico.

Treatment

- Curative treatments for localized, good, and intermediate prognostic groups are radical prostatectomy, conformal radiotherapy to the prostate, and brachytherapy. Sometimes a "watch and wait policy" is proposed.
- Patients with poor prognostic characteristics are likely to receive external radiotherapy with androgen deprivation therapy (ADT) or even palliative transurethral resection (TUR) and ADT.
- Metastatic disease is treated first by ADT, but all tumors progress to castration-refractory prostate cancer (CRPC). The standard treatment of CRPC is chemotherapy, particularly docetaxel, which induces a significant increase of median survival and a decrease of pain and analgesic consumption. Other palliative symptomatic treatments are useful.

There are neither prospective studies aimed to establish standard treatment in senior adult prostate cancer patients nor specific guidelines for the treatment of this patient population. However, retrospective studies have been performed in the setting of both localized and metastatic disease. The International Society of Geriatric Oncology (SIOG) Prostate Cancer Task Force has prepared recommendations for the management of senior adult prostate cancer patients (Droz JP et al. 2010, Droz JP et al. in press). These are used as a basis for the following recommendations for patient management.

Treatment of Localized Prostate Cancer in Senior Adult Patients

Evidence suggests that only a minority of senior adults with localized prostate cancer receive curative therapy. The 2008 EAU guidelines recommend that "as a standard, an assessment of the patient's life expectancy, overall health status and tumor characteristics is necessary before any treatment decision can be made." It is also stated that "life expectancy, rather than patient age, should be the factor considered in treatment selection." Panel members did not select a specific chronological cutoff point for treatment recommendations.

- Alibhai and colleagues have evaluated treatment efficacy in men aged ≥65 years with localized prostate cancer by using a decision model that integrates the patient's age, comorbidity, Gleason score, patient preference, and treatment efficacy data (from three complementary data sources including modern radiotherapy results). Their results show that prostatectomy and radiotherapy significantly improve life expectancy and quality-adjusted life expectancy in older men with little comorbidity and moderately or poorly differentiated localized prostate cancer. As healthy men in their 70s or 80s with localized prostate cancer are often managed conservatively, they conclude that "curative therapy should be seriously considered in men up to age 80 years who have high-grade disease."
- Retrospective and cohort studies have demonstrated that the presence of comorbidities in patients receiving a prostatectomy significantly and independently increases the risks of 30-day postoperative complications, long-term incontinence, and overall and nonprostate cancer death. However, the risk of incontinence is known to increase proportionally with age. It is therefore recommended to limit the indication of prostatectomy to patients less than 75 years old.
- Several studies have reported that senior adult patients undergoing radiotherapy can achieve outcomes in terms of cancer control and

treatment-related late comorbidity similar to those achieved by younger patients. A population-based study of nonmetastatic prostate cancer patients aged 65 to 85 years treated with radiotherapy has shown improved long-term survival rates for patients with locally advanced stage receiving adjuvant ADT but no survival advantage for men with low-risk disease. These findings are consistent with practice guidelines. However, the survival advantage achieved by combining radiotherapy and ADT in high-risk prostate cancer patients may apply only to those with no or minimal comorbidities (i.e., fit patients).

- Brachytherapy is indicated in patients with low-risk prostate cancer. This technique does not appear to be a suitable treatment choice for older prostate cancer patients because its clinical benefit is not established.
- Older prostate cancer patients are more likely to be eligible for a "watch and wait" policy.

The SIOG Task Force conclusion was as follows:

- Treatment decisions should be based on patient's actual health status (mainly dependent on the severity of associated comorbid conditions) rather than on chronological age, and also on patient preference.
- "Fit" and "vulnerable" senior adults in the "high-risk" group of the D'Amico risk classification with a chance of surviving >10 years are likely to benefit from curative treatment.
- Senior adults in the "low-risk" and "intermediate-risk" groups of the D'Amico risk classification are likely to benefit from active surveillance.

Treatment of Metastatic Prostate Cancer in Senior Adult Patients

- ADT is the standard treatment for patients with metastatic prostate cancer. It delays progression, prevents potentially catastrophic complications, and effectively palliates symptoms. Surgical castration and castration by luteinizing hormone–releasing hormone agonists (LHRHa) are the standard of care. ADT is associated with a significant number of side effects, including osteopenia with increased risk of fractures, and metabolic alterations with increased risk of cardiovascular events.

⊐ Bone mass decreases with age, and men ≥75 years of age are at particularly high risk of developing fractures. The National Comprehensive Cancer Network (NCCN) recommendations state that men receiving or starting ADT should be evaluated for risk of osteoporosis.

- All men receiving ADT should receive calcium and vitamin D supplementation, and baseline bone mineral density should be determined.
- The routine use of bisphosphonates in patients undergoing ADT is not recommended unless there is documented evidence of the presence or a risk of osteoporosis or CRPC with skeletal metastases.

- The standard procedure for second-line hormonal treatment is as follows:
  ⊐ Cessation of ADT if given as first-line treatment in association with an LHRHa
  ⊐ The addition of an antiandrogen when the LHRHa was used as monotherapy in the first-line setting
- Docetaxel is the only palliative treatment that has demonstrated a survival benefit in patients with CRPC. In subgroup analyses, the survival benefit with thrice-weekly docetaxel is consistent between age classes (<65 years, ≥65 years, and ≥75 years). The tolerability of the thrice-weekly docetaxel regimen has not been specifically studied in frail senior adults. The place of weekly docetaxel in metastatic CRPC should be further evaluated.
- Other palliative treatments include palliative surgery, radiopharmaceuticals, radiotherapy, and medical management of pain and symptoms.

Conclusion

Senior adult patients with prostate cancer should be managed according to their individual health status, which is mainly related to the severity of associated comorbid conditions and not to chronological age. Evidence-based medicine guidelines must be applied in senior adults with prostate cancer, together with guidelines used for younger patients. Therefore, the standard and universally accepted EAU guidelines should be adhered to. Nevertheless, their application must be modified according to the actual

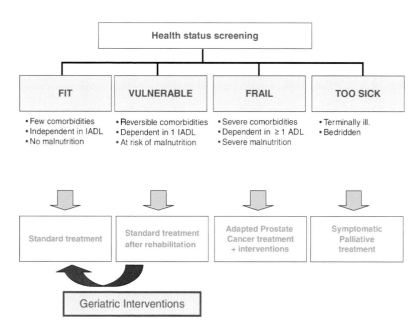

ADL: Activity of Daily Living; IADL: Instrumental ADL.

Figure 1 *Principles of the decision tree (International Society of Geriatric Oncology Prostate Cancer Task Force).*

health status of each individual patient. Figure 1 shows how treatment could be adapted using a simplified health status evaluation.

Acknowledgments

The authors thank Marie-Dominique Reynaud for edition of the manuscript.

Declaration of Interest:

Dr Droz has reported that he is a member of the speaker's bureau for Sanofi-Aventis and Novartis.

Dr Terret has not reported any conflicts of interest.

Dr Fléchon has not reported any conflicts of interest.

Further Reading

Alibhai SM, Naglie G, Nam R, et al. Do older men benefit from curative therapy of localized prostate cancer? J Clin Oncol 2003; 21:3318–3327.

Berthold DR, Pond GR, Soban F, et al. Docetaxel plus prednisone or mitoxantrone plus prednisone for advanced prostate cancer: updated survival in the TAX 327 study. J Clin Oncol 2008; 26:242–245.

D'Amico AV, Moul J, Carroll PR, et al. Cancer-specific mortality after surgery or radiation for patients with clinically localized prostate cancer managed during the prostate-specific antigen era. J Clin Oncol 2003; 21:2163–2172.

Droz JP, Balducci L, Bolla M, et al. Background for the establishment of SIOG guidelines for the management of prostate cancer in senior adults. Crit Rev Hemat Oncol 2010; 73:68–91.

Droz JP, Balducci L, Bolla M, et al. SIOG guidelines for the management of prostate cancer in older men: recommendations of a working group of the International Society of Geriatric Oncology. BJU Int in press.

Heidenreich A, Aus G, Bolla M, et al. EAU guidelines on prostate cancer. Eur Urol 2008; 53:68–80.

National Comprehensive Cancer Network. NCCN clinical practice guidelines in oncology: senior adult oncology v.1.2009. Available at: http://www.nccn.org/professionals/physician_gls/f_guidelines.asp. Accessed June 2009.

Bladder Cancer

M. Maffezzini and F. Campodonico
Department of Urology, E.O. Ospedali Galliera, Genoa, Italy

Incidence and Mortality

Bladder cancer (BC) ranks fourth among solid tumors accounting for about 7% of all cancers. In Europe, the estimated incidence is 136,000 cases per year. The annual incidence rate is 22/100,000 men and 4/100,000 women, and the corresponding mortality rate is 7/100,000 and 2/100,000, respectively. BC is fatal in about one-third of men and one half of women, thus explaining the social interest of the disease. The frequency of diagnoses reaches a peak at 65 years of age, and two-thirds of BC patients are older than 65 years. Since the average age of the population is increasing, the incidence of BC is expected to increase accordingly.

Etiology and Risk Factors

Tobacco smoking is responsible for 65% of all cases of BC in the male and 30% in the female population. The relative risk (RR) of developing BC in smokers is two to four times that of nonsmokers. Aromatic amines includingnaphtylamines, and specifically, benzidines, and derivatives, are likely to be involved in tobacco smoking as well as in the occupational environment (i.e., industrial manufacturing of chemicals, hair dyes, rubber, metal).

Pathology

BC is constituted by transitional cell carcinoma (TCC) in about 90% of cases. Urothelial cancer is used as a synonym. About 90% of TCCs are observed in the urinary bladder, 8% in the renal pelvis or calyx, and the remaining 2% within the ureter. Less frequently, the urothelial lining of the urethra can also be a site of disease. Adenocarcinoma, squamous cell carcinoma, and small cell carcinoma account for the remaining 10% of histotypes.

Natural History and Tumor Biology

At presentation the disease is limited to the mucosa, submucosal layer, or lamina propria of the bladder in about 75% of cases, referred to as non-muscle-invasive bladder cancer (NMIBC). Infiltration into the muscular wall is present in the remaining cases. In about 50% to 80% of cases, the disease shows an intrinsic tendency toward recurrence. Progression to muscle-invasive disease, chiefly depending on grade and stage of initial lesion/s, can be observed in up to 50%.

BC is likely to represent two distinct diseases.

- A low-risk or low-grade papillary malignancy that rarely invades or metastasizes
- A less common high-risk disease with high-grade lesions invasive from the onset (about 15–25% of cases), with a high tendency to invasion, that frequently metastasizes and can be fatal

Low-grade, noninvasive, and high-grade invasive represent the two ends of a spectrum of diseases, however, BC can also show the ability to progress from one end of the spectrum to the other or intermediate risk.

Peculiar features are shown by carcinoma in situ or Cis or Tis. It consists of a poorly differentiated flat, intraepithelial lesion. Macroscopically, its recognition is inconstant. When visible, it is represented by velvety spots, reddish in color. Cis can be found in association with established high-grade, invasive, and also with nonmuscle infiltrative disease. Although its natural history is incompletely understood, the presence of Cis bears a substantially negative influence on prognosis.

Signs and Symptoms

Macroscopic, asymptomatic hematuria is the most frequent and only sign of BC. Vesical irritation alone, lower urinary tract symptoms, or prostatism in the male, can be the only presenting symptom associated with Cis.

Imaging, Cystoscopy, and Urinary Cytopathology

Although ultrasonography is used in the initial evaluation, in the presence of gross or microscopic hematuria, an intravenous pyelogram (IVP) is indicated. Abdomen and pelvic computed tomography (CT) scans with contrast medium are often used as substitutes for IVP bearing in mind that underestimation and overestimation of the infiltration of the bladder wall occur in up to 50%.

Tumors of the urothelium exfoliate cells in the urine, therefore, urinary cytopathology (UC) is of help especially in the diagnosis of lesions not detectable at cystoscopy (Cis).

Staging

The most widely accepted staging classification is the TNM system (UICC 2002).

T or primary tumor
Tx primary cannot be assessed.
T0 no evidence of primary.
Ta noninvasive, limited to the mucosa.
Tis, also Cis, flat tumor limited to the mucosa (high grade).
T1 noninvasive, infiltration of the basal membrane and limited to the subepithelial connective tissue.
T2 muscle invasive, T2a inner half, T2b, outer half.
T3 invasion of the perivesical fat; T3a, microscopic invasion; T3b, gross invasion.
T4 invasion of neighboring structures; T4a, prostate, uterus, vagina; 4b, pubis, muscles of the pelvic/abdominal wall.

N or regional nodes
The nodes located within the true pelvis are considered as regional lymph nodes.
Nx no information on nodal status.
N0 no evidence of tumor within the nodes examined.
N1 tumor present in one node and ≤ 2 cm in maximum diameter.
N2 metastasis in a single node >2 cm but <5 cm in greatest diameter or multiple nodes <5 cm.
N3 lymph node metastasis >5 cm.

M or distant metastasis
Mx no information on M.
M0 absence of distant metastasis.
M1 distant metastasis.

Histopathologic grading (G)
GX grade not assessed.
G1 well differentiated.
G2 moderately differentiated.
G3–4 poorly differentiated.

Additional descriptors include lymphatic vessel invasion (L) and venous invasion (V).

Accurate pathological diagnosis, grading, and staging of BC represent the cornerstone for treatment strategy.

Treatment of NMIBC

Transurethral resection of bladder (TURB) represents the only modality that allows for accurate diagnosis, grading, and staging of the disease. The superficial portion of the lesion/s and the underlying muscular wall are sampled and sent separately to the pathologist as "endoluminal" portion and a full-thickness sample of the detrusor muscle underlying the tumor. Absence of orientation may negatively affect the accuracy of stage definition.

TURB also constitutes standard treatment for NMIBC when complete eradication of all visible lesions is obtained. Morbidity and mortality after TURB are low, and five-year survival is high, however, local control of disease is achieved in less than one-third of the patients.

- TURB alone is recommended in patients in the low-risk category.
- TURB with intravesical instillation with topical antitumor agents is recommended for intermediate-risk patients.
- TURB with intravesical instillation of Bacillus Calmette Guerin (BCG) is recommended in patients at high risk.

Laser treatment, and fulguration are considered palliative treatments.

Surgical Treatment

Radical cystectomy (RC) is standard treatment for muscle-invasive disease, as well as for recurrent NMIBC stages Cis, or pTis, pT1 G3. RC includes the ablation of the bladder en bloc with the prostate and seminal vesicles in the male patient, and bladder, uterus, ovaries, and a portion of the anterior vaginal wall in the female patient.

Bilateral pelvic lymphadenectomy is considered part of the procedure, although the boundaries of lymph node removal are currently under debate.

The increasing age of the population has led to an increased diagnosis of muscle-infiltrative BC also in the elderly. Cancer treatment has been underresearched in the older population, and with regard to BC, age and comorbidity constitute a bias against both clinical trials and standard treatments as well. In population-based studies, only 1 man in 6 aged 75 years receives RC for MIBC, and 1 in 10 receives RC for MIBC at the age of 80 years. Because of refinements in patient selection in the elderly and in perioperative management, RC is considered also in aged subjects.

Urinary diversion encompasses several possibilities ranging from the simple ureterocutaneostomy and ureteroileostomy to more sophisticated forms of urinary diversion consisting in continent reservoirs obtained from intestinal segments. Such reservoirs can be implanted at the anatomical site of the native bladder, referred to as orthotopic neobladders. Alternatively, continent catheterizable reservoirs can be implanted at a different site, most frequently the lower right abdomen, and are referred to as heterotopic reservoirs. Indications for each type of urinary diversion are based on the features both of the tumor and of the host, generally leaving the simplest forms for locally advanced, poor prognosis tumors in surgically unfit patients and the more complex continent reconstruction for good prognosis tumors in fit patients.

Complications of RC and urinary diversion are reported in the range of 15% to 35% of cases mainly influenced by general patients status and complexity of diversion.

Partial cystectomy consists in the surgical removal of a portion of the bladder harboring BC It should be restricted to poor anesthesiology risk candidates for palliative purposes.

Radiotherapy

Radical radiotherapy is considered as a treatment option for patients with major contraindications for surgery. Although the optimal tumoricidal dose is unknown, most recent series recommend the dose of 65 Gy.

Organ-Sparing Treatments

Organ-sparing treatments have been explored with the purpose to maintain the native bladder in muscle-invasive BC. This includes, TURB and chemo- and/or radiotherapy.

Chemotherapy (CT) is used at reduced doses as radiosensitizer, after TURB, in association with external beam irradiation. Five-year survival similar to RC has been reported in the relatively limited number of studies available, and the bladder is retained in about 40% of patients treated with this approach. Local toxicity of the combined treatments in some patients may represent a cause of cystectomy.

Organ-sparing treatment is considered as investigational treatment.

Systemic Chemotherapy

Systemic CT has been used for MIBC in combination with surgery as neoadjuvant before RC or as adjuvant following RC. There are several limitations of the published trials: heterogeneity of criteria of eligibility, long time of recruitment (a decade or more), premature closure, lack of statistical power, differences in definitive treatment (RC or RT), and number of dropout cases. However, a meta-analysis showed a limited survival advantage, around 5%, in favor of neoadjuvant platinum-based CT.

Systemic CT constitutes the treatment of choice for advanced, metastatic disease, and platinum should constitute the backbone of CT combinations.

Prognosis of BC

Tumor recurrence and progression are the clinically relevant events associated with the diagnosis of NMIBC. Generally, pTa and pT1 tumors have a good prognosis with low lethal potential, whereas Tis or Cis tends to behave aggressively. Tumor recurrences and new occurrences are observed in approximately two-thirds of patients during follow-up depending on several acknowledged prognostic factors such as stage, grade, number, and size of initial lesions. The presence of recurrence at the first three-months cystoscopy is a strong predictor of prognosis. Progression of disease, that is, the risk of developing muscle invasion from initially noninvasive lesions also varies depending on stage, grade, number, and size of initial lesion/s from approximately 4% for low-grade Ta tumors to 50% for high-grade T1 tumors. Associated Cis is known to increase substantially the risk of progression.

The five-year survival after RC for MIBC is generally unsatisfactory. It varies from 40% to 60% for stage pT2 N0 M0 to around 15% for stage pT4. Survival for pN positive patients may vary from 6 to 24 months from surgery.

Follow-Up

The follow-up schedule is based on what is known of the natural history of the disease or, in other words, on the risk of progression.

- Patients with pTa, pT1, and low-grade tumors should receive UC and cystoscopy three to four times per year for the first two years and at six-month intervals for the following three years.
- Patients with high-grade lesions or Cis should be followed at three-month intervals for the first three years and at six-month intervals thereafter.

The follow-up after RC should monitor the potential sites of recurrence, namely, the urethra and the pelvis, as well as upper urinary urothelium, liver, lungs, and skeletal apparatus.

Declaration of Interest:

Dr Maffezzini has not reported any conflicts of interest.

Dr Campodonico has not reported any conflicts of interest.

Further Reading

Audisio RA, Pope D, Ramesh HS, et al. Shall we operate?: Preoperative assessment in elderly cancer patients (PACE) can help: a SIOG surgical task force prospective study. Crit Rev Oncol Hematol 2008; 65:156–163.

Maffezzini M, Campodonico F, Canepa G, et al. Current peri-operative management of radical cystectomy with intestinal urinary reconstruction for muscle-invasive bladder cancer and reduction of postoperative ileus. Surg Oncol 2008; 17:41–48.

Raghavan D, Suh T. Cancer in the elderly population. The protection racket. J Clin Oncol 2006; 24:1–2.

Stenzl A, Cowan NC, De Santis M, et al. The updated EAU guidelines on muscle-invasive and metastatic bladder cancer. Eur Urol 2009; 55:815–825.

Gynecological Cancer in the Senior Patient

17

W.A.A. Tjalma

*Department of Gynaecological Oncology & University
Multidisciplinary Breast Clinic Antwerpen, University Hospital
Antwerpen, Antwerp (Edegem), Belgium*

Introduction

About 20% of visceral cancers in women are of the genital tract. The top three genital tract malignancies are uterine, ovarian, and cervical cancers. The lifetime risk of developing these cancers in an industrialized country is respectively 1 in 38, 1 in 68, and 1 in 135. Unfortunately, many women are not treated according to the guidelines, which results in a poor survival. A lack of surgical skills is the main reason. This chapter gives an overview of the different treatment strategies for local, locoregional, and metastatic genital tract cancers in senior women.

Cervical Cancer

The staging of cervical cancer is clinically based on the Fédération internationale de Gynécologie Obstétrique (FIGO) staging system. The squamous carcinomas account for 80% of all cases and are declining due to the screening. The adenocarcinomas account for 15%, but the incidence has almost doubled the last 20 years despite screening.

The diagnosis is made by a (cone) biopsy. The average age of a women with cervical cancer is between 35 and 45. The 2008 FIGO staging system is used.

Stage 0 Cervical Cancer

This is carcinoma in situ. The five-year survival rate is 100%. Treatment could be conisation (preferable) or hysterectomy. One can opt for the latter if the patient has other gynecological problems.

Stage I Cervical Cancer

This is cancer strictly confined to the cervix, and it can be divided into IA and IB. The five-year survival is about 80%. Surgery for these patients is the preferred approach. However, if the patient is unfit for surgery, one can opt for concomitant chemoradiation or radiotherapy alone.

Stage IA1

This stage includes tumors with stromal invasion of ≤ 3 mm in depth and horizontal extension of ≤ 7 mm. Adenocarcinomas and adenosquamous carcinomas should be treated in the same way as squamous carcinomas.

- If there is no lymphovascular space invasion (LVSI), the preferred treatment is conisation or type 1 hysterectomy if there are associated (benign) problems. There is no indication for node dissection (lymph node metastasis rate is <0.5%) or ovariectomy.
- If there is LVSI, the preferable treatment in elderly women is a type 1 or 2 hysterectomy with pelvic node dissection. A node dissection is indicated since the lymph node metastasis rate is up to 4.7%. There is no indication for an ovariectomy. An alternative for a hysterectomy could be a conization or modified radical trachelectomy.

Stage IA2

This stage includes tumors with a stromal invasion of >3 mm and ≤ 5 mm in depth and horizontal extension of ≤ 7 mm.

- If there is no LVSI, the rate of lymph node metastasis is up to 3.4%. The treatment could be conisation or a type 1 hysterectomy or sometimes a radical trachelectomy or a type 2 hysterectomy. All procedures should be combined with a pelvic (laparoscopy/laparotomy) node dissection. There is no indication for an ovariectomy.
- If there is LVSI, the rate of lymph node metastasis is up to 11.1%. The treatment options are radical trachelectomy with laparoscopic pelvic lymph node dissection or a type 2 hysterectomy with pelvic node dissection. There is no indication for an ovariectomy.

Stage IB1

This is a clinically visible lesion ≤4.0 cm in greatest dimension.

- One should opt for a type 2 or 3 hysterectomy. The operation should always be combined with a bilateral pelvic lymphadenectomy. Alternatively a radical trachelectomy, either vaginal or abdominal, can be performed. The radical trachelectomy should ideally be reserved for patients with a well-differentiated tumor of less than 2 cm in size and no evidence of LVSI.
- Another approach is concomitant chemoradiation therapy.

Stage IB 2

This is a clinically visible lesion >4.0 cm. The treatment can be a type 2 or 3 radical hysterectomy with bilateral pelvic and para-aortic lymph node dissection or concomitant chemoradiation.

Primary concomitant chemoradiation [cisplatin 40 mg/m^2/wk intravenously during radiotherapy (six weeks)] is equally effective as primary radical surgery for disease-free and overall survival. Treatment choice is based on the features of the tumor, the treatment-related morbidity, condition, and wishes of the patient. One should try to avoid the combination of chemoradiation and radical surgery to reduce therapy-related morbidity.

Patients with lymph node metastasis or positive tumor margins should receive adjuvant concomitant chemoradiation. Ideally, only radical surgery should be performed on patients with no lymph node involvement. The sentinel node biopsy could be ideal to tailor the treatment. The technique is feasible, but its sensitivity and specificity are unclear at the moment. Studies are ongoing to evaluate the value of sentinel node biopsy in patients with cervical cancer. Until the results are known, sentinel node biopsy cannot be considered as the standard approach for patients with cervical cancer.

Stage II

Tumor extends beyond the cervix but not to the pelvic sidewall nor to the lower third of the vagina. The five-year survival is 60%.

Stage II is subdivided into the following:

- IIA tumor: no parametrial involvement
  - ⌐ IIA1: clinical lesion ≤4.0 cm
  - ⌐ IIA2: clinical visible lesions >4.0 cm

  Treatment in the same way as stage IB
- IIB tumor: with obvious parametrial involvement

  Treatment: concomitant chemoradiation is the preferred approach.

Stage III

The tumor extends to the pelvic sidewall and/or the lower one-third of the vagina and/or causes hydronephrosis or a nonfunctioning kidney. Overall survival is 30%.

Stage III is subdivided into the following:

- IIIA: Tumor involves lower third of the vagina, with no extension to the pelvic wall.
- IIIB: Extension to the pelvic wall and/or hydronephrosis or nonfunctioning kidney.

  The preferred treatment is concomitant chemoradiation.

Stage IV

Tumor extends beyond the true pelvis or involves (biopsy proven) the mucosa of the bladder or rectum. A bullous edema, as such, does not permit a patient to be allotted to stage IV. Overall survival is 5%.

It is subdivided into the following:

- IVA: spread of growth to adjacent organs

  Standard treatment is concomitant chemoradiation. If there are fistula or if it is only localized disease with no signs of disease outside the pelvis, one can opt for pelvic exenteration. However, this leads to a high morbidity, and a careful staging is of utmost importance.

- IVB: spread to distant organs

  Treatment is palliative and consists of chemotherapy. Chemotherapy (e.g., cisplatin, carboplatin, paclitaxel, or topotecan) can give a response in up to 30% of patients.

Uterine Cancer

Uterine cancer is the most common malignancy of the female tract in the industrialized world. Its incidence in women less than 65 years is 13.1/100,000 and in women over 65 years 98.5/100,000. The incidence worldwide is 17.8/100,000. The 2008 FIGO staging system is used.

Stage I

In stage I the tumor is confined to the uterine corpus. The five-year survival is about 90%.

Stage I can be divided into the following:

- IA: No or less than half of the myometrium is invaded.

  Treatment consists of hysterectomy with bilateral salpingo-oophorectomy; lymph node dissection should be considered if the tumor is ≥grade II. In patients with papillary serous or clear cell carcinoma histology, a lymph node dissection should also be performed.

- IB: Invasion to equal or more than half of the myometrium.

  The preferred treatment is a hysterectomy with bilateral salpingo-oophorectomy with pelvic and para-aortic lymph node dissection.

Adjuvant radiotherapy is indicated in case of lymph node involvement. Adjuvant chemotherapy is probably as effective as radiotherapy in early endometrial cancers. In patients with papillary serous or clear cell carcinoma, the preferred treatment is carboplatin in combination with paclitaxel.

Stage II

In stage II the tumor invades the cervical stroma but does not extend beyond the uterus. The five-year survival is between 70% and 80%. Treatment is similar to that for stage IB.

Stage III

In this stage there is local and/or regional spread of the tumor. Positive cytology has to be reported separately without changing the stage. The five-year survival is about 30% to 60%.

Stage III can be divided into the following:

- IIIA: Tumor invades the serosa of the corpus uteri and/or adnexae.
- IIIB: Vaginal and/or parametrial involvement.
- IIIC: Metastases to pelvic and/or para-aortic lymph nodes.
    - IIIC1: Positive pelvic nodes.
    - IIIC2: Positive para-aortic lymph nodes with or without positive pelvic lymph nodes.

    Treatment is similar to stage IV disease.

Stage IV

In stage IV the tumor invades bladder and/or bowel mucosa, and/or distant metastases are present. The five-year survival is about 10%.

Stage IV can be divided into the following:

- IVA: tumor invasion of bladder and/or bowel mucosa
- IVB: distant metastases, including intra-abdominal metastases and/or inguinal lymph nodes

Stages III and IV are best treated by optimal cytoreductive surgery followed by systemic chemotherapy and/or radiotherapy. Chemotherapy regimens should preferably include doxorubicin and cisplatin or carboplatin and paclitaxel. When there is widespread metastatic disease and the tumor is estrogen receptor and/or progesterone receptor positive, hormonal therapy (progestins, tamoxifen, or aromatase inhibitor) should be considered. This can be alone or following chemotherapy.

Pelvic exenteration should be considered occasionally when the tumor is limited to the bladder or rectum.

Special Types of Endometrial Malignancy

About 3% of endometrial malignancies are sarcomas. Uterine sarcomas can be classified as leiomyosarcoma, endometrial stromal sarcoma, high-grade undifferentiated sarcoma (HGUD), or pure heterologous sarcoma. The 2008 FIGO staging system is used.

Carcinosarcomas

Carcinosarcomas should be staged as carcinomas of the endometrium.

The treatment of leiomyosarcomas, endometrial stromal sarcomas, and adenosarcomas consists of a hysterectomy without lymph node dissection (Tables 1 and 2). A bilateral salpingo-oophorectomy is recommended for postmenopausal women. No adjuvant therapy is indicated.

In advanced stages of leiomyosarcomas, chemotherapy and/or hormonal therapy should be used. The endometrial stromal sarcomas and adenosarcomas are preferably treated with hormonal therapy.

Vaginal Cancer

Primary vaginal cancers represent only 2% of female genital tract malignancies. It is mainly a disease of women older than 60 years. Women treated for anogenital precancerous lesions or cancer in the past are considered high risk for vaginal cancer. The 2008 FIGO staging system is used.

Stage 0

Stage 0 represents a carcinoma in situ. The five-year survival is 100%. The preferred treatment is surgical excision of the lesion.

Stage I

In stage I the disease is limited to the vagina wall. The five-year survival in 70%.

The preferred treatment is an excision of the lesion (so-called partial or complete vaginectomy) and lymph node dissection.

- If the lesion is in the upper one-third of the vagina, it should be pelvic lymphadenectomy.
- If the lesion is located in the lower one-third part, an inguinal lymphadectomy should be performed.
- If the lesions are located in the middle, both inguinal and pelvic lymphadnectomy should be performed.

Sentinel node biopsy will be helpful in determining which nodes should be removed, but at present there are no data supporting the use of this

Table 1 *Leiomyosarcomas and Endometrial Stromal Sarcomas[a]*

Stage I	Tumor limited to uterus
IA	≤5.0 cm
IB	>5.0 cm
Stage II	Tumor extends beyond the uterus, within the pelvis
IIA	Adnexal involvement
IIB	Involvement of other pelvic tissues
Stage III	Tumor invades abdominal tissues (not just protruding into the abdomen)
IIIA	One site
IIIB	>one site
IIIC	Metastasis to pelvic and/or para-aortic lymph nodes
Stage IV	
IVA	Tumor invades bladder and/or rectum
IVB	Distant metastasis

[a]Simultaneous endometrial stromal sarcomas of the uterine corpus and ovary/pelvis in association with ovarian/pelvic endometriosis should be classified as independent tumors.

Table 2 *Adenosarcomas*

Stage I	Tumor limited to uterus
IA	Tumor limited to endometrium/endocervix with no myometrial invasion
IB	Less than or equal to half myometrial invasion
IC	More than half myometrial invasion
Stage II	Tumor extends beyond the uterus, within the pelvis
IIA	Adnexal involvement
IIB	Involvement of other pelvic tissues
Stage III	Tumor invades abdominal tissues (not just protruding into the abdomen)
IIIA	One site
IIIB	>one site
IIIC	Metastasis to pelvic and/or para-aortic lymph nodes
Stage IV	
IVA	Tumor invades bladder and/or rectum
IVB	Distant metastasis

procedure, and because of the rareness of the disease, it is unlikely that there will be any data to support the use of sentinel node biopsy in vaginal cancer.

Concomitant chemoradiation can be used as an alternative to surgery.

Stage II

In stage II the carcinoma involves the subvaginal tissue but has not extended to the pelvic wall. The five-year survival is 50%. The treatment is similar to that for stage I disease.

Stage III

In stage III the carcinoma has extended to the pelvic wall. The five-year survival is 20%. If possible, surgery can be considered; however, the preferable treatment in this stage is concomitant chemoradiation.

Stage IV

In stage IV the carcinoma has extended beyond the true pelvis or has involved the mucosa of the bladder or rectum; bullous edema, as such, does not permit a patient to be allotted to stage IV.

Stage IV can be divided into the following:

- IVA: Tumor invades bladder and/or rectal mucosa and/or direct extension beyond the true pelvis.

  Treatment: In localized disease, a pelvic exenteration is a surgical option with a cure rate of about 50%.
- IVB: Spread to distant organs.

  Treatment: Palliative chemotherapy can be considered.

The prognosis of stage IV disease is poor, with a five-year survival of <10%. However, in case of a rectovaginal or vesicovaginal fistula with distant disease, one should also consider exenteration or derivation surgery to improve quality of life.

Adjuvant concomitant chemoradiation is recommended in case of lymph nodes or surgical margin involvement.

Vulvar Cancer

Primary vulvar cancers represent about 4% of female genital tract malignancies. It is mainly a disease for women older than 60 years. The 2008 FIGO staging system is used.

Stage 0

Stage 0 represents a carcinoma in situ. The five-year survival is 100%. The preferred treatment is surgical excision of the lesion. Alternatively, after invasive disease has been ruled out, topical administration of 5-fluorouracil or imiquimod can be used.

Stage I

In stage I the tumor is confined to the vulva.

Stage I can be divided into the following:

- IA: The lesions are ≤2.0 cm in size, confined to the vulva or perineum and with stromal invasion <1.0 mm and no nodal metastasis(es).

  Treatment consists of wide local excision (tumor-free margin ≥1.0 cm) without lymph node dissection.
- IB: The lesions are >2.0 cm in size or with stromal invasion ≥1.0 mm, confined to the vulva or perineum with negative nodes.

  Treatment consists of wide local excision or (hemi)vulvectomy (tumor-free margin ≥1.0 cm) with lymph node dissection.
    - ⌐ The use of sentinel node biopsy is recommend for evaluation of the lymph nodes.
        - If the lymph node is involved, an inguinofemoral lymphadenectomy should be performed.
            - ○ For centralized lesions, a bilateral inguinofemoral lymphadenectomy is indicated.
            - ○ For lateralized lesion, an ipsilateral iguinofemoral lymphadenectomy is performed.
    - ⌐ Adjuvant chemoradiation is indicated in patients with involved lymph nodes or margins, which cannot be reresected. Preferably, cisplatin is used as a radiation sensitizer.

Stage II

Stage II consists of a tumor of any size with extension to adjacent perineal structures (one-third of lower urethra, one-third of lower vagina, anus) without lymph node involvement.

Treatment is similar to that for stage IB.

Stage III

Stage III encompasses a tumor of any size with or without extension to adjacent perineal structures (one-third of lower urethra, one-third of lower vagina, anus) with involvement of inguinofemoral lymph nodes.

Stage II can be divided into the following:

- IIIA: (*i*) one or two lymph node metastasis(es) (<5.0 mm) or (*ii*) one lymph node metastasis (≥5.0 mm)
- IIIB: (*i*) three or more lymph node metastases (<5.0 mm) or (*ii*) two or more lymph node metastases (≥5.0 mm)
- IIIC: positive lymph nodes with extracapsular spread

  The treatment should be individualized. In selected patients, radical vulvectomy with bilateral inguinofemoral lymphadenectomy is indicated, which is sometimes preceded by neoadjuvant chemotherapy and postoperative radiotherapy. All other patients should be treated by chemoradiation.

Stage IV

In stage IV the tumor invades other regional (two-thirds of upper urethra, two-thirds of upper vagina) or distant structures.

It can be divided into the following:

- IVA: Tumor invades any of the following: (*i*) upper urethral and/or vaginal mucosa, bladder mucosa, rectal mucosa, or fixed to pelvic bone or (*ii*) fixed or ulcerated inguinofemoral lymph nodes.

  Treatment: See stage III. In cases of fistualisation or centralized local disease, a exenteration can be considered.

- IVB: Any distant metastasis(es) including pelvic lymph nodes.

  Treatment consists of palliative chemotherapy (e.g., cisplatin, carboplatin, paclitaxel, or topotecan) and can result in a response in up to 20% of patients.

Ovarian Cancer, Fallopian Tube Cancer, and Primary Peritoneal Cancer

For staging of ovarian and primary peritoneal cancer, the FIGO 1988 staging system is used, while for fallopian tube cancer, the 1991 system is used. The majority of women (70%) are diagnosed in an advanced stage (III/IV). The five-year survival for these stages is <50% (Tables 3 and 4).

Treatment

Borderline Tumors

The treatment should only consist of a surgical resection of the tumor and implants. There is no role for lymphadenectomy or adjuvant chemo- or radiotherapy.

Invasive Ovarian and Peritoneal Cancers

Patients with invasive cancers should have a meticulous surgical staging. The staging includes an en bloc resection of the ovarian tumor and the other ovary, hysterectomy, pelvic and para-aortic lymphadenectomy, omentectomy, aspiration of free fluid or peritoneal washings, and systematic exploration of the lower and upper abdomen with removal of all adhesions or suspicious lesions. In mucinous tumors, an appendectomy should also be performed.

The goal of surgery is the removal of all visible lesions (optimal debulking or cytoreductive surgery = no visible residual disease). If this cannot be achieved, the value of surgery is minimal. Unfortunately, many women are suboptimally debulked.

When the preoperative evaluation indicates that the patient cannot be optimally debulked because of lack of surgical skills or extensive disease or when the patient is in a poor surgical condition, one should opt for neo-adjuvant chemotherapy. In case of a response allowing optimal surgery,

Table 3 Staging of Ovarian Cancer

Stage I	Growth limited to the ovaries
IA	Growth limited to one ovary; no ascites present containing malignant cells. No tumor on the external surface; capsule intact.
IB	Growth limited to both ovaries; no ascites present containing malignant cells. No tumor on the external surfaces; capsules intact.
IC	Tumor either stage IA or IB, but with tumor on surface of one or both ovaries or with capsule ruptured or with ascites present containing malignant cells or with positive peritoneal washings.
Stage II	Growth involving one or both ovaries with pelvic extension.
IIA	Extension and/or metastases to the uterus and/or tubes.
IIB	Extension to other pelvic tissues.
IIC	Tumor either stage IIA or IIB, but with tumor on surface of one or both ovaries or with capsule(s) ruptured or with ascites present containing malignant cells or with positive peritoneal washings.
Stage III	Tumor involving one or both ovaries with histologically confirmed peritoneal implants outside the pelvis and/or positive regional lymph nodes. Superficial liver metastases equals stage III. Tumor is limited to the true pelvis, but with histologically proven malignant extension to small bowel or omentum.
IIIA	Tumor grossly limited to the true pelvis, with negative nodes but with histologically confirmed microscopic seeding of abdominal peritoneal surfaces or histologic proven extension to small bowel or mesentery.
IIIB	Tumor of one or both ovaries with histologically confirmed implants, peritoneal metastasis of abdominal peritoneal surfaces, not exceeding 2.0 cm in diameter; nodes are negative.
IIIC	Peritoneal metastasis beyond the pelvis >2.0 cm in diameter and/or positive regional lymph nodes.
Stage IV	Growth involving one or both ovaries with distant metastases. If pleural effusion is present, there must be positive cytology to allot a case to stage IV. Parenchymal liver metastasis equals stage IV.

Table 4 *Staging of the Cancer of the Fallopian Tube*

Stage 0	Carcinoma in situ (limited to tubal mucosa).
Stage I	Growth limited to the fallopian tubes.
IA	Growth is limited to one tube, with extension into the submucosa and/or muscularis but not penetrating the serosal surface; no ascites.
IB	Growth is limited to both tubes, with extension into the submucosa and/or muscularis but not penetrating the serosal surface; no ascites.
IC	Tumor either stage IA of IB, but with tumor extension through or into the tubal serosa or with ascites present containing malignant cells or with positive peritoneal washings.
Stage II	Growth involving one or both fallopian tubes with pelvic extension.
IIA	Extension and/or metastasis to the uterus and/or ovaries.
IIB	Extension to other pelvic tissues.
IIC	Tumor either stage IIA of IIB and with ascites present containing malignant cells or with positive peritoneal washings.
Stage III	Tumor involves one or both fallopian tubes, with peritoneal implants outside the pelvis and/or positive regional lymph nodes. Superficial liver metastasis equals stage III. Tumor appears limited to the true pelvis, but with histologically proven malignant extension to the small bowel or omentum.
IIIA	Tumor is grossly limited to the true pelvis, with negative nodes, but with histologically confirmed microscopic seeding of abdominal peritoneal surfaces.
IIIB	Tumor involving one or both tubes, with histologically confirmed implants of abdominal peritoneal surfaces, none exceeding 2.0 cm in diameter. Lymph nodes are negative.
IIIC	Abdominal implants >2.0 cm in diameter and/or positive retroperitoneal or inguinal nodes.
Stage IV	Growth involving one or both fallopian tubes with distant metastases. If pleural effusion is present, there must be positive cytology to be stage IV. Parenchymal liver metastases equals stage IV.

interval debulking surgery should be performed. Sometimes palliative surgery is performed to improve the quality of life.

Adjuvant chemotherapy therapy should be given to all patients with stage IA (grades II and III), IB (grade II and III), IC, II, III, and IV. The combination of carboplatin with paclitaxel is the first choice. It can be administrated intravenously or in selected patients intraperitoneally.

Relapse of Ovarian and Peritoneal Cancers

The majority of patients will relapse. The relapse time is important for determining treatment. If the disease relapses after one year of primary therapy, the initial medication can be used again. If the disease relapses within one year, other drugs should be used. These other drugs include single-agent or combination therapy of liposomal doxorubicin, gemcitabine, topotecan, hexamethylmelamine, or oral etoposide. Alternatively, one can opt for tamoxifen (hormonal therapy) or bevacizumab (monoclonal antibody therapy). Secondary cytoreductive surgery should only be performed after response to chemotherapy and if the surgeon thinks that optimal debulking can be achieved.

Conclusion

Selected gynecological cancers are mainly observed in senior patients, and for many, cancer surgery is the main treatment option. Senior patients should receive the same treatment as younger women if their surgical condition allows optimal surgery. The multimodality treatment of gynecological malignancies should be considered in fit senior patients, but interdisciplinary cooperation is of utmost importance to select the appropriate treatment for the individual senior patient.

Declaration of Interest:

Dr Tjalma has reported no conflicts of interest.

Further Reading

Bouchardy C, Rapiti E, Blagojevic S, et al. Older female cancer patients: importance, causes, and consequences of undertreatment. J Clin Oncol 2007; 25:1858–1869.

Head and Neck Cancer in the Elderly

18

E.M. Karapanagiotou
*Athens School of Medicine, Sotiria General Hospital, Athens,
Greece; and The Royal Marsden Hospital NHS Foundation Trust, London, U.K.*

K.J. Harrington
The Royal Marsden Hospital NHS Foundation Trust, London, U.K.

K.N. Syrigos
Athens School of Medicine, Sotiria General Hospital, Athens, Greece

Introduction

Squamous cell carcinoma of the head and neck (SCCHN) represents the sixth most common malignancy. The usual age of diagnosis is between the fifth and sixth decades, but as many as 24% of SCCHN are diagnosed in patients older than 70 years of age. There are no major differences in terms of disease stage and tumor differentiation between senior and younger patients, although the elderlies present a trend to develop more locally advanced disease but fewer neck node metastases. Radiotherapy (RT) and surgery or both combined represent the principal treatment modalities, but chemotherapy and targeted therapies also play a central role in disease management in senior patients.

Surgery

The majority of retrospective studies support surgery as the treatment of choice if the primary tumor can be excised with an appropriate margin of normal tissue without causing major functional compromise. This treatment modality can be as effective in senior patients as in younger patients without a significant increase in mortality and complications. An aggressive approach to SCCHN with adoption of a curative intent can also be considered in elderly patients with advanced cancer.

The presence of comorbidities represents the key indicator for a senior patient selected for surgical management, since they influence not only the administration of anesthesia but also the incidence of postoperative complications.

Reconstructive surgery with free flaps in the elderly is a controversial area because of the presence of degenerative conditions and comorbidities. However, several retrospective studies show that it is a safe and reliable option.

The choice of local therapy should take into account the following:

- The likely functional outcome of treatment
- The resectability of the tumor
- The comprehensive geriatric assessment
- The patient's wishes

Radiotherapy

RT for SCCHN can be delivered with curative intent (radical RT) to improve local control following surgery (adjuvant RT) or to provide symptomatic relief (palliative RT). RT alone results in high tumor control and cure rates for early-stage glottic and oropharyngeal cancers. Moreover, by default, it represents the treatment of choice for those who are considered unfit for surgery or in whom surgery would lead to unacceptable functional outcome.

RT is effective and well tolerated in the ageing population with SCCHN, and undoubtedly, age does not represent a limiting factor for radiation therapy. The most widely used RT fractionation in senior patients is conventional fractionation of 1.8 to 2.0 Gray (Gy)/fraction five days a week over seven weeks. There is no consensus whether altered fractionation is better than conventional RT with curative intent in SCCHN. A meta-analysis of 15 randomized trials with 6515 patients showed that altered fractionation is better than conventional RT for overall survival and primary tumor control, but there was a suggestion of a decreasing effect of altered fractionation RT with increasing age and poor performance status (PS). Senior patients showed lower compliance and tolerance, besides there being an excess in non-cancer-related deaths in patients over 71 years old.

Regarding acute and late toxicities, they do not seem to differ between younger and elderly patients, although older patients suffer more functional mucositis and therefore may suffer increased weight loss and electrolyte disturbances.

Chemotherapy

Chemotherapy is administered concomitantly with RT for locoregional disease or in the palliative setting for recurrent locoregional or metastatic disease. Chemoradiation is also beneficial in the postoperative setting when extracapsular spread or positive margins are present. Multiagent induction chemotherapy administered before definitive chemoradiation seems to offer remarkable response rates as well as reduction of distant metastases.

- Combined data from two mature phase III randomized studies (ECOG 1393 and ECOG 1395) showed that patients aged 70 years or older had similar objective response rates and median time to progression compared with younger patients but at a cost of significant nephrotoxicity, diarrhea and thrombocytopenia. A higher rate of toxic deaths was noted in the elderly but did not reach statistical significance.
- The Meta-Analyses of Chemotherapy in Head and Neck Cancer (MACH-NC), where 87 trials and 16,665 patients were included between 1965 and 2000, showed that the benefit of adding chemotherapy to locoregional treatment is significantly decreasing with increasing age. The proportion of deaths not related to SCCHN increased with age from 15% at age 50 years to 39% at age ≥ 71 years. On the basis of these data, chemotherapy is generally administered in patients aged <71 years old.

Age has been associated with pharmacokinetic and pharmacodynamic changes and with increased susceptibility of normal tissues to toxic complications. Chemotherapy complications such as neutropenia, anemia, bleeding, mucositis, cardiac toxicity, and neurotoxicity are more frequently observed in the elderly and may precipitate a loss of functional independence.

Targeted Therapies

The immunoglobulin (Ig)G1 monoclonal antibody against the ligand domain of epidermal growth factor receptor (EGFR), cetuximab, has been approved for concurrent administration with radical external beam RT in locoregionally advanced SCCHN as well as in combination with platinum-based chemotherapy as first-line treatment in patients with recurrent or metastatic disease. There are no clinical studies with sufficient numbers of senior patients (65 years and over) with SCCHN testing cetuximab to determine whether they respond differently from younger patients. Cetuximab is safely administered in the elderly, but the experience is limited in patients 75 years of age and above. There is a consensus for administering cetuximab to senior patients with renal or hearing impairment or poor PS concomitantly with RT in locally advanced disease where cisplatin administration is contraindicated. Patients older than 65 years or with poor PS do not benefit in terms of overall survival if cetuximab is added to platinum-based chemotherapy.

Conclusion

Medical intervention in the elderly is justified when the potential benefits outweigh the potential risks. There is almost complete consensus that patients suffering from operable squamous cell cancer of the head and neck area should be treated with curative intent if thorough preoperative assessment of comorbidities is performed. Age does not represent a limiting factor for RT delivery but altered fractionation seems to be beneficial only for patients aged <71 years old. Patients aged ≥71 years old do not benefit from chemotherapy added to locoregional therapy. Targeted therapies play an important role in combination with external beam radiation in locally advanced disease.

Declaration of Interest:

Dr Syriogos has not reported any conflicts of interest.

Dr Karapanagiotou has not reported any conflicts of interest.

Dr Harrington has not reported any conflicts of interest.

Further Reading

Bourhis J, Overgaard J, Audry H, et al. Hyperfractionated or accelerated radiotherapy in head and neck cancer: a meta-analysis. Lancet 2006; 368:843–854.

Pignon JP, Maitre A, Bouhris J, on behalf of the MACH-NC Collaborative Group. Meta-analyses of chemotherapy in head and neck cancer (MACH-NC): an update. Int J Radiat Oncol Biol Phys 2007; 69(2 suppl):S112–S114.

Syrigos KN, Karachalios D, Karapanagiotou EM, et al. Head and neck cancer in the elderly: an overview on the treatment modalities. Cancer Treat Rev 2009; 35:237–245.

Zabrodsky M, Calabrese L, Tosoni A, et al. Major surgery in elderly head and neck cancer patients: immediate and long-term surgical results and complication rates. Surg Oncol 2004; 13:249–255.

Renal Cell Cancer

J. Bellmunt

*Department of Medical Oncology, University Hospital del
Mar-IMIM, Barcelona, Spain*

Introduction

Renal cell carcinoma (RCC) primarily affects older individuals, with approximately half of all new RCC diagnoses being made in persons 65 years of age or older and an incidence of 56 per 100,000 persons. Epidemiological studies have described that up to two-thirds of 75-year-olds with renal cancer suffer from conditions such as hypertension, cardiovascular disease, or diabetes. Gastrointestinal disorders are also frequent in these patients.

Several of the novel, targeted agents are associated with toxicities such as hypertension or diarrhea, which have especial relevance to an elderly population. Drugs taken to manage comorbid conditions (such as antihypertensives and oral anticoagulants) may interact with agents given to treat malignancies, altering pharmacokinetics and potentially increasing toxicity, reducing efficacy, or both. Furthermore, in patients with cognition impairment, some side effects of targeted agents (e.g., fatigue, diarrhea, and dehydration) are exacerbated and may result in delirium. Fatigue and asthenia are another frequently observed and clinically significant side effect of targeted agents in senior adult patients. Physical therapy may be a suitable preventive intervention in patients who experience these symptoms.

It should be emphasized that although toxicity is not always more frequent in the elderly population than in younger patients, its impact may be greater. Therefore, agents commonly associated with these side effects should be carefully monitored and, if used, particular attention should be given to the dose used and additional supportive measures such as hydration and support from a caregiver.

Surgery in the Senior Cancer Patient

The potential risks and benefits of cytoreductive nephrectomy in elderly renal cancer patients have been compared with those of a younger group. In both age groups, 79% of patients had distant metastases. The study confirmed the additional surgical risk in patients aged over 75 years: perioperative mortality (i.e., within a month of surgery) was 21% (5 deaths in 24 patients), compared with 1% in a large cohort of younger patients with similar disease characteristics and performance status. Early mortality in the elderly was associated with longer surgery time and greater blood loss, which, the investigators suggest, puts unsustainable strain on diminished physiological reserves. However, even when these early deaths were included, the median overall survival (OS) among patients aged over 75 was 16.6 months. This was not significantly different from the 13.7-month median OS in younger patients, although it should be noted that the number of patients involved in the study was small.

Given the limited amount of information, it would be appropriate to comment that patients aged over 65 years are more likely to encounter postoperative complications. Although selected patients undoubtedly do well, the decision to undertake cytoreductive nephrectomy should be approached with caution. This is perhaps especially so now that targeted therapies are available, since the role for nephrectomy in these changed circumstances has still to be demonstrated.

Systemic Therapy of Metastatic Renal Cell Carcinoma in the Senior Cancer Patient

Until recently, treatment options were limited for elderly patients with RCC. Options for the medical management of metastatic RCC (mRCC) have been radically improved through the introduction of agents targeting tumor angiogenesis or intracellular pathways mediating growth and proliferation. Recommendations are needed on how to integrate specific management strategies into clinical practice that will optimize the use of these agents in the elderly. The goal is to maximize the clinical benefit with strategies focused on patient selection, assessment of quality of life, management of adverse events, and appropriate dose modifications.

Principal among targeted agents are the small-molecule inhibitors sorafenib (Nexavar®), sunitinib (Sutent®), everolimus (Afinitor®), temsirolimus (Torisel®), and the monoclonal antibody bevacizumab (Avastin®).

- Sorafenib and sunitinib are orally bioavailable, small-molecule tyrosine kinase inhibitors (TKIs). They have a broad range of targets, among which they both inhibit vascular endothelial growth factor (VEGF) and platelet-derived growth factor (PDGF) receptor tyrosine kinases.
- Temsirolimus and everolimus differ from these agents in targeting mammalian target of rapamycin (mTOR) that belongs to a cell growth and proliferation pathway frequently activated in advanced renal cell cancers.
- The monoclonal antibody bevacizumab has antiangiogenic activity by targeting different isoforms of vascular endothelial growth factor (VEGF).

All these targeted agents have been shown to add significant clinical benefit when compared with placebo or interferon (IFN) therapy in the treatment of mRCC (Table 1). Even though at present, it does not seem that targeted agents will offer a complete cure for mRCC with careful management, they may offer the potential to transform mRCC into a chronically treatable disease. Indeed, the median OS for patients with mRCC has increased from around 13 months in the immunotherapy era to around 24 to 26 months in more recent years.

Randomized controlled trials (RCTs) show that five targeted agents—sorafenib, sunitinib, temsirolimus, bevacizumab, and everolimus—improve outcome in advanced RCC. Pazopanib is a new player in mRCC based on the results presented at ASCO 2009. However, physicians need to be aware of particular considerations when choosing a treatment regimen for their elderly patients with RCC.

Clinical experience suggests that the toxicities associated with sorafenib, sunitinib, and bevacizumab-INF are different and it may be helpful to take this into account in the case of individual patients (such as those who have cardiac risk factors or are elderly). Given the data available from randomized trials, sunitinib—along with bevacizumab plus INF (see later)—should be considered the preferred first-line therapy in patients at good and intermediate risk, although sorafenib (no supporting randomized

Table 1 *Summary of Phase III Clinical Trials with Targeted Agents*

Trial designs	Line of treatment/ patient characteristics	Benefit from novel agent
Sorafenib vs. placebo	Second line/ECOG 0–1	Median PFS 5.5 vs. 2.8 mo
		Better OS (censoring data for crossover)
Sunitinib vs. IFN	First line/ECOG PS 0–1	Median PFS 11 vs. 5 mo
		Median OS 26 vs. 22 mo[a]
Bevacizumab plus IFN vs. placebo plus IFN	First line	Median PFS 10.2 vs. 5.4 mo
Bevacizumab plus IFN vs. IFN	First line	Median PFS 8.5 vs. 5.2 mo
Temsirolimus vs. IFN	First line (poor risk)	Median OS 11 vs. 7 mo[b]
Everolimus vs. placebo	Second line post TKI	Median PFS 4.0 vs. 1.9 mo

[a]Significant when patients crossing over from IFN to sunitinib are excluded.
[b]Comparison is temsirolimus versus IFN; median OS in the temsirolimus plus IFN arm was eight months.
Abbreviations: IFN, interferon; PFS, progression free survival; PS, performance status; TKI, tyrosine kinase inhibitor; OS, overall survival; mo, months; ECOG, Eastern Cooperative Oncology Group.
Source: From Bellmunt J, Négrier S, Escudier B, et al. Crit Rev Oncol Hematol 2009; 69:64–72.

data) might be indicated in selected populations at risk. Everolimus is approved in the European Union (EU) and the United States for the treatment of advanced RCC that has progressed on or after treatment with VEGF-targeted therapy.

None of the phase III trials listed in Table 1 had an upper age limit to recruitment. This itself is of interest, since a maximum age would generally have been stipulated in similar studies carried out a decade ago. Across these studies and their treatment arms, the average age of patients entered was remarkably similar (the lowest median being 58 years in the sorafenib arm of the placebo-controlled phase III and the highest a median of 62 years in the sunitinib arm of the study vs. IFN). These trials were also very consistent in the range of ages included (typically, the youngest patients entered were 25–35 years old, and the most elderly 80–86 years). Along the same lines, recent pivotal trials in mRCC are notable for the fact that they have not restricted eligibility by age. All included some patients over the age of 80 years, and around a third of those accrued were aged over 65.

This offers the opportunity for subgroup analyses to assess the relationship of age with treatment benefit. Since such analyses have been undertaken retrospectively, they should be regarded as hypothesis generating and certainly not as definitive. Nevertheless, they provide grounds for further investigation. All the recent randomized phase III trials report the proportion of patients aged 65 years or over: 36% in the sunitinib study, 30% in the sorafenib study, 30% in that involving temsirolimus, and 37% in the bevacizumab trial. This proportion—roughly one-third—certainly under-represents the proportion of patients aged over 65 years in the general population of patients with mRCC. However, since these trials were large, there were sufficient elderly patients involved to allow at least some assessment of the relationship between age and the efficacy and tolerability of treatment.

While these trials were similar in age characteristics, they differ somewhat in the apparent effect of age on the benefits of treatment.

- The sunitinib and bevacizumab studies suggest that the effect of these targeted agents is little—if at all—influenced by age.
- In the sorafenib study, however, it seems that the benefit of this TKI relative to placebo is greater in more elderly patients than in the younger group.
- Hazard ratios from the subset analysis of the temsirolimus study suggest a trend toward the reverse effect, but confidence intervals around these estimates are wide and no definite conclusion can be drawn on this point without a prospective study (Fig. 1).

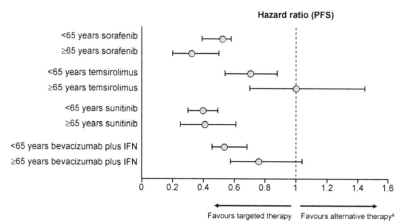

Figure 1 Progression-free survival benefit of targeted therapies in elderly and younger patients enrolled in phase III clinical trials. Sorafenib versus placebo; temsirolimus, sunitinib, and bevacizumab plus IFN versus IFN. Abbreviation: IFN, interferon.

Patient-Focused Approach

The populations enrolled in the pivotal RCTs differs, and to date, no head-to-head comparisons allow us to judge relative efficacy and tolerability. Patients with mRCC represent an heterogeneous group, and no one agent will provide optimal benefit to all patients. In addition, populations recruited to RCTs underrepresent certain patient subtypes, notably the elderly and those with comorbidities. Consequently, the suitability of a specific targeted agent for a given patient group, such as the elderly, will depend on a number of factors, including disease-, patient- and treatment-related characteristics. Data from expanded access studies and clinical experience may be as relevant as the results of RCTs when making this difficult decision.

To show how different sources of data can be integrated, a schema has been proposed, which acknowledges nine factors relevant to clinical decision-making and provides an easily understandable visual indication when assigning the strength with which a particular agent can be recommended for use in specific subgroups of patients (Fig. 2). In this "patient-focused schema," an individualized approach to treatment selection is proposed. Treatment should be tailored according to the available agent (sunitinib,

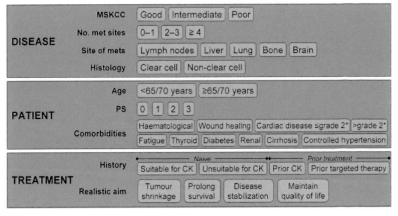

DISEASE	MSKCC	Good	Intermediate	Poor		
	No. met sites	0–1	2–3	≥ 4		
	Site of mets	Lymph nodes	Liver	Lung	Bone	Brain
	Histology	Clear cell	Non-clear cell			
PATIENT	Age	<65/70 years	≥65/70 years			
	PS	0	1	2	3	
	Comorbidities	Haematological	Wound healing	Cardiac disease ≤grade 2*	>grade 2*	
		Fatigue	Thyroid	Diabetes	Renal	Cirrhosis	Controlled hypertension
TREATMENT	History	Naive	Suitable for CK	Unsuitable for CK	Prior treatment	Prior CK	Prior targeted therapy
	Realistic aim	Tumour shrinkage	Prolong survival	Disease stabilization	Maintain quality of life	

* Including controlled arrhythmias.

CK=cytokines; mets=metastases; MSKCC=Memorial Sloan-Kettering Cancer Center; No.= number of; PS = performance status; RCC = renal cell carcinoma.

Figure 2 *Parameters to consider when choosing an appropriate treatment for the individual patient with renal cell cancer. Including controlled arrhythmias. Abbreviations: CK, cytokines; met, metastasis; MSKCC, Memorial Sloan-Kettering Cancer Center; No., number of; PS, performance status.*

sorafenib, bevacizumab, temsirolimus, everolimus) to meet individual circumstances and needs. For a given case, patient-, disease-, and treatment-related characteristics should be evaluated individually. These should be taken into consideration together with the efficacy and toxicity/ tolerability profile of each targeted agent to allow a tailored treatment.

We recommend the integration of this approach into everyday clinical practice, even though achieving this is a considerable clinical challenge. Notably, more recently published international guidelines for the treatment of RCC, such as the kidney cancer guidelines of the National Comprehensive Cancer Network (NCCN), recognize the importance of an individualized approach to therapy and base their recommendations on broader criteria, emphasizing the value of clinical judgment and experience to support treatment decisions for individual patients.

In the absence of controlled comparisons between them, it is not possible to say that any of the agents reviewed is more or less suited to use in elderly patients in general. Even indirect comparison of the relative frequency or severity of a specific toxicity is inappropriate since the phase III studies, which provide the most robust toxicity data, were conducted in different populations and the side effects of treatment were assessed by different groups of investigators. However, considering the ranking of toxicities as they appeared for each agent in the pivotal phase III studies (Table 2) might

Table 2   Most Common Adverse Events (All Grades) in Descending Order of Frequency, as Reported in Three Pivotal Studies with Single-Agent Targeted Therapy

Sorafenib	Sunitinib	Temsirolimus
Nonhematological		
Diarrhea	Diarrhea	Asthenia
Rash or desquamation	Fatigue	Rash
Fatigue	Nausea	Nausea
Hand-foot skin reaction	Stomatitis	Anorexia
Alopecia	Vomiting	Pain
Nausea	Hypertension	Dyspnea
Pruritis	Hand-foot syndrome	Infection
Hypertension	Mucosal inflammation	Diarrhea
Anorexia	Rash	Peripheral edema
Vomiting	Asthenia	Cough
Hematological		
Decreased hemoglobin	Leukopenia Neutropenia	Anemia Thrombocytopenia
Other laboratory abnormalities		
None listed	Increased creatinine Increased lipase	Hyperlipidemia Hyperglycemia

Source: From Bellmunt J, Négrier S, Escudier B, et al. Crit Rev Oncol Hematol 2009; 69:64–72.

be reasonable when assessing treatment options in an individual patient with comorbidities. Besides, this should be suited together with the "patient-focused schema." A definitive answer to the question of whether drugs should be selected according to specific comorbidities will require prospectively designed trials.

Conclusion

Many elderly patients require special considerations when devising a treatment plan. Age-related physiological, cognitive, and social characteristics seen in this patient population may influence patient selection, goals of treatment, response to therapy, and the management of adverse effects. None of these factors, however, should necessarily preclude an elderly patient from treatment with targeted therapies. With a proper understanding of these particular considerations, appropriate preparation and patient education, and regular monitoring for and management of adverse effects, elderly patients with RCC can benefit from targeted therapies.

Declaration of Interest:

Dr Bellmunt has reported that he is a member of the Advisory Board for Bayer Health Care, Pfizer, Novartis and Roche. He is also a consultant for Bayer Health Care and Pfizer.

Further Reading

Bellmunt J, Flodgren P, Roigas J, et al. Optimal management of metastatic renal cell carcinoma: an algorithm for treatment. BJU Int 2009; 104:10–18.

Bellmunt J, Mulders P, Szczylik C, et al. Defining a new patient-focused treatment approach to renal cell carcinoma (RCC). Ann Oncol 2008; 8:197.

Bellmunt J, Negrier S, Escudier B, et al. The medical treatment of metastatic renal cell cancer in the elderly: position paper of a SIOG Taskforce. Crit Rev Oncol Hematol 2009; 69:64–72.

Coebergh JW, Janssen-Heijnen ML, Post PN, et al. Serious co-morbidity among unselected cancer patients newly diagnosed in the southeastern part of The Netherlands in 1993-1996. J Clin Epidemiol 1999; 52:1131–1136.

Kader AK, Tamboli P, Luongo T, et al: Cytoreductive nephrectomy in the elderly patient: the M. D. Anderson Cancer Center experience. J Urol 2007; 177: 855–860; discussion 860–861.

Psychological Problems in Older Cancer Patients

M.I. Weinberger
Department of Psychiatry, Weill Cornell Medical College,
White Plains, New York, U.S.A.

E.M. Balk, C.J. Nelson, and A.J. Roth
Department of Psychiatry and Behavioral Sciences, Memorial Sloan-Kettering
Cancer Center, New York, New York, U.S.A.

Introduction

Depression and anxiety are two of the most prevalent psychological disorders in older cancer patients. Given the severity of a cancer diagnosis, it is understandable for patients to experience symptoms of general distress, worry, and anxiety. However, distress is often experienced on a continuum from minor situational anxiety and transient depressive symptoms to more severe disorders that require intervention and treatment. Throughout the cancer experience, patients may have brief periods of denial or despair followed by distress, with a mixture of depressed mood and anxiety, insomnia, and irritability. These symptoms may last for days to several weeks, after which usual patterns of adaptation return. This response is highly variable, however, it is important to remember that consistent symptoms of severe depression or anxiety are not part of a normal adjustment process for older patients with cancer.

Depression

Despite the high prevalence rates and deleterious effects of depression, elderly patients are far less likely to be diagnosed with major depression or dysthymia than any other age group. Moreover, when depression is present, it is frequently undertreated.

Depressive symptoms manifest themselves differently in both later adulthood and in patients with cancer. For example, the symptoms of cancer and the side effects of treatment such as pain, fatigue, insomnia, changes in appetite, anxiety, or adjustment to the cancer diagnosis often overlap with many symptoms of depression. Older depressed adults often present with more somatic complaints (such as body aches and malaise) as opposed to affective complaints (i.e., sadness, guilt, and self-criticism). The prevalence of depression in patients with cancer has ranged from 6% to 25%.

Many cancer centers now screen patients for general psychological distress using the distress thermometer, a brief self-administered visual analog scale that has been used extensively and well validated in patients with cancer. This tool may be a good gateway for more elaborate screening for anxiety and depression.

Depression in Geriatric Patients with Cancer

Exploration of the two gateway symptoms of depression is important (i.e., depressed mood and loss of interest). It is important to elicit information about other potential symptoms of depression in older patients. These would include "general malaise" as opposed to being depressed or having loss of interest due to pain or fatigue, or "general" aches and pains or stomach aches as opposed to specific tumor site pain or specific side effect of cancer treatment. Hopelessness is also an important aspect to investigate; many patients with cancer express some hope for a meaningful future regardless of prognosis, or a cure of their cancer; thus reporting little or no hope for either may be a sign of depression. Sleep may be problematic for both patients with cancer and older patients; however, it is important to ask if the patient wakes up in the middle of the night (middle insomnia) and has difficulty getting back to sleep because they worry or feel anxious or wake up too early in the morning. An older depressed patient may also report mood variation during the day.

Treatment for Depressed Patients with Cancer

While there is evidence about the efficacy of treatments for geriatric depression, there is minimal evidence specifically demonstrating the effectiveness of psychological and pharmacologic treatments in depressed patients with cancer. The level and duration of distress, the inability to carry out daily activities, and the response to psychotherapeutic interventions are the signs used to determine when a psychotropic medication is needed.

- Medications that are typically used to treat depression in patients with cancer are those that are used in treating depression in general. Most commonly, serotonin-specific reuptake inhibitors (SSRIs) and serotonin-norepinephrine reuptake inhibitors (SNRIs) are prescribed for older patients with cancer. All antidepressants now carry a 'Black Box' warning for possibly causing suicidal ideation.
  - ⅂ The SSRIs do not have the same risks of cardiac arrhythmias, hypotension, and troublesome anticholinergic effects such as urinary retention, memory impairment, sedation, and reduced awareness as do older antidepressants such as the tricyclic antidepressants (TCAs). The most common side effects of the SSRIs include gastric distress and nausea, brief periods of increased headache, and insomnia (and sometimes hypersomnia). Some patients may experience anxiety, tremor, restlessness, and akathisia, while others may feel sluggish. SSRIs can cause sexual dysfunction in men and women, a side effect that often leads to cessation of the medication even in older adults. Consideration must be given to interactions with other medications such as coumadin, digoxin, and cisplatin.

    All the SSRIs have the ability to inhibit the hepatic isoenzyme P450 2D6. It is important to consider additional drug-drug interactions especially in the elderly who may be on multiple medication regimens and have various physicians. This has been elucidated as many antidepressants decrease effective levels of tamoxifen, a hormonal agent used in breast cancer. It appears that venlafaxine and mirtazapine are least interactive with tamoxifen, though further research is needed. SSRIs should be avoided with the chemotherapeutic agent procarbazine, which has monoamine oxidase inhibitor (MAOI)-like properties.
  - ⅂ SNRIs are potent inhibitors of neuronal serotonin and norepinephrine reuptake. They are similar to TCAs in terms of efficacy, without the same problematic side effects. These antidepressants should also not be used in patients receiving MAOIs. Mirtazapine is a sedating antidepressant, useful in depressed patients with associated anxiety and insomnia. It has few gastrointestinal and sexual side effects and may induce weight gain. It is usually dosed at bedtime because it can be sedating.

- Bupropion has an activating side effect profile that makes it useful in lethargic medically ill patients, yet it should be avoided in patients with a history of seizure disorders and in those who are malnourished; it may cause anxiety or restlessness in some patients.
- TCAs may be used when patients have severe, treatment-resistant depression or have concomitant neuropathic pain syndromes; however, they are difficult for the elderly to tolerate at therapeutic doses. The anticholinergic actions of TCAs can cause confusion as well as serious tachycardia, and the quinidine-like effects of TCAs can lead to arrhythmias. Postural hypotension and dizziness may also occur; these are of particular concern for the frail, volume-depleted patient who is at risk for falls and possible osteoporosis-related fractures. Urinary retention and constipation are also problematic side effects for the elderly.
- Psychostimulants may be used when there is coexisting fatigue or malaise. There is growing experience for supporting the use of these medications to treat depressive symptoms in patients with cancer on the basis of their quick response time and its alleviation of concomitant symptoms of fatigue, sedation, and poor concentration. They may be useful early in the treatment of depression until an antidepressant has a chance to become therapeutic.

Choosing an antidepressant in the elderly cancer population may be based on whether a patient or a family member has responded well to an antidepressant in the past. Other factors that should be considered include the patient's overall health and cognitive abilities; the social and financial resources, which are often limited in this patient population; and any other existing psychiatric conditions (i.e., substance abuse, psychosis, or anxiety disorders). Additionally, it is useful to note if there is a need for physical symptom control (i.e., neuropathic pain, fatigue, and insomnia) as well as management of the psychiatric symptoms. It is helpful to consider the side effect profiles of different antidepressants that may be useful as well as those that should be avoided. For example, if a patient presents with fatigue or sedation, the most appropriate agent may be an energizing antidepressant or a psychostimulant. Consider mirtazapine in a patient who is experiencing anxiety or insomnia, gastric upset, or loss of appetite.

Patients who are unable to swallow pills may be able to take an antidepressant in an elixir or mirtazapine, which comes in a soluble tablet preparation. Patients with stomatitis secondary to chemotherapy or radio-therapy or those who have slow intestinal motility or urinary retention should receive an antidepressant with the least anticholinergic side effects.

Psychotherapy, including supportive therapy, psychoeducational inter-ventions, cognitive behavioral therapy (CBT), interpersonal therapy (IPT), and problem-solving therapy also appear to help older depressed patients with cancer. Supportive techniques such as active listening with supportive comments can be readily applied by oncologists and oncology nurses. Cognitive therapy, which focuses on how an individual's inaccurate thoughts or assessments of his/her situation lead to anxious and depressed feelings, can be used to help a patient develop an adaptive perspective on his/her circumstances.

- CBT has been found to help depressed patients with cancer, in particular by combining behavioral activation with cognitive techniques.
- Group therapy for patients with cancer, caregivers, and families may be advantageous, allowing individuals to receive support from others facing similar problems.

Anxiety

Anxiety disorders in older cancer patients are common. As with depression, there needs to be greater attention on understanding and recognizing anxiety disorders in older adults with cancer.

Anxiety in Geriatric Patients with Cancer

Prevalence rates of anxiety vary between 1% and 23% in studies of patients with cancer. In patients with advanced cancer, rates of anxiety have been found to be close to 30%. Older adults with cancer often have multiple medical conditions and complex polypharmacy issues that may blur the clinical presentation of anxiety. The diagnosis of anxiety in older patients with cancer is usually determined by questions about ongoing worry, restlessness, pacing, apprehension, and hypervigilance. Several factors that can complicate the diagnosis of anxiety in older patients with cancer include pain, respiratory distress, sepsis, endocrine abnormalities, hypoglycemia, hypocalcemia, hormone-secreting tumors, and pancreatic cancer. A change in metabolic state or an impending medical catastrophe may be heralded by symptoms of anxiety. Suddenly occurring symptoms of anxiety with chest pain, respiratory distress, restlessness, and a feeling of "jumping out of my skin" may indicate a pulmonary embolus. Patients who are hypoxic often appear anxious and fear that they are suffocating or dying.

The use of steroids, antiemetics, and withdrawal from narcotics, benzodiazepines, and alcohol can all cause anxiety. Akathisia, a common side effect of neuroleptic drugs used to control nausea, may often manifest as anxiety and restlessness. These symptoms can be controlled by the addition of a benzodiazepine or a β-blocker.

Withdrawal states from alcohol, opioids, and benzodiazepines are often overlooked as causes of anxiety and agitation even in older patients. Patients in the palliative care setting may have been prescribed shorter-acting benzodiazepines (e.g., lorazepam, alprazolam, and oxazepam) to control both anxiety and nausea. With inadequate dosing or tapering regimens, these patients often have rebound anxiety or withdrawal between doses.

Panic disorder often presents as a sudden, unpredictable episode of intense discomfort and fear with thoughts of impending doom. Patients who have already compromised respiratory function may have cyclical exacerbations of their anxiety and breathing problems. Symptoms of a preexisting panic disorder may intensify during the palliative care phase when patients are confronting increasing physical symptoms and disability and their own mortality.

Treatment for Anxious Older Patients with Cancer

Psychotherapeutic and pharmacologic approaches have been shown to successfully treat anxiety disorders in older adults. Individual and group cognitive-behavioral interventions and supportive therapy, IPT, problem-solving therapy, and insight-oriented therapy have been used successfully with older patients to relieve anxiety.

- For patients with mild to moderate anxiety, the use of psychological techniques alone may be sufficient to assist them in managing anxiety. Psychoeducational interventions are particularly useful for anxious patients who have difficulty understanding medical information about their prognoses and symptoms. Explaining the predictable emotional phases through which patients pass as they face new and frightening information may also alleviate their anxiety. Providing information to patients' families enables them to cope more effectively, which in turn enhances patients' sense of support. Cognitive-behavioral interventions include reframing negative, irrational thought processes, progressive relaxation, distraction, guided imagery, meditation, biofeedback, and hypnosis. Other psychotherapeutic techniques such as supportive and insight-oriented therapy may be helpful to reduce anxiety symptoms and allow for better coping with the cancer. When working with older cancer patients, having the flexibility to adjust the length of sessions, intervals between sessions, and use of the telephone for those who have difficulty coming into your office is imperative.

- One quarter to one-third of patients with advanced cancer receive antianxiety medication during their hospitalizations. In deciding whether a pharmacological approach may be useful, the severity of the patient's anxiety symptoms and the degree to which they interfere with overall well-being are the most reliable guides. Given the possibility of compromised hepatic and renal functioning, as well as increased sensitivity to pharmacological interventions, if drugs are to be used in older patients, the rubric of starting with lower doses than would be used with younger, physically healthy patients, and increasing these doses more cautiously will lead to more successful outcomes.

  ⌐ The first-line antianxiety drugs are the benzodiazepines. In older patients, however, these medications may result in mental status changes such as confusion or impaired concentration or memory. These changes are more often seen in those with advanced disease and those with impaired hepatic or brain function. Dose-dependent side effects such as drowsiness, confusion, and decreased motor coordination must be monitored carefully in elderly patients. Benzodiazepine use represents an important iatrogenic risk factor for falls for older adults. One must keep in mind the synergistic effects of the benzodiazepines with other medications that have central nervous system (CNS) depressant properties such as narcotics and some antidepressants. Elderly patients with dementia or brain injury who are administered benzodiazepines may experience paradoxical behavioral disturbances such as aggressiveness, irritability, and agitation.

  ⌐ For insomnia, the benzodiazepine temazepam as well as the non-benzodiazepine hypnotics zolpidem, zaleplon, eszopiclone, or ramelteon may be effective. In addition, sedating antidepressants such as trazodone or mirtazapine may also help patients with persistent anxiety and insomnia. A sedating atypical neuroleptic such as olanzapine or quetiapine may be effective for the patient who is anxious or has trouble sleeping and is confused or has respiratory compromise. Neuroleptics may also be useful for the patient whose anxiety is substance induced (e.g., steroids) or in anxious patients with severely compromised pulmonary function. Buspirone is useful for patients with generalized anxiety disorder and for those in whom there is the potential for abuse. Buspirone is not effective on an as-needed basis, and its effects are not apparent for one to two weeks.

⌐ In the oncology setting, the SSRIs are effective in the management of generalized anxiety and panic disorder.

Conclusions

Anxiety and depression are highly prevalent in older patients with cancer. This chapter has provided a summary of the issues that need to be considered when diagnosing and treating older cancer patients with anxiety and depression. Diagnosing depression and anxiety in older patients with cancer is difficult. Therefore, clinicians need to be familiar with the unusual presentation of these symptoms in this population.

Psychotherapeutic and psychopharmacological interventions are optimal in treating anxiety and depression in older patients with cancer. Oncologists should be aware of the indications for psychotropic medications, the possible side effects and drug interactions of psychiatric medications, and how to obtain psychiatric consultation when needed.

Declaration of Interest:

Dr Roth, Dr Weinberger, Dr Balk, and Dr Nelson have reported no conflicts of interest.

Further Reading

Extermann M, Hurria A. Comprehensive geriatric assessment for older patients with cancer. J Clin Oncol 2007; 25:1824–1831.

Roth A, Modi R. Psychiatric issues in older cancer patients. Crit Rev Oncol Hematol 2003; 48:185–197.

Weinberger MI, Roth AJ, Nelson CJ. Untangling the complexities of depression diagnosis in older cancer patients. Oncologist 2009; 14:60–66.

Social and Ethical Aspects

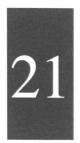

G.B. Zulian

Department of Rehabilitation and Geriatrics, University Hospitals of Geneva, Geneva, Switzerland

Introduction

In our westernized society, about three-quarters of citizen will eventually become senior adults, meaning they have reached at least the age of 70 years. They will have raised their family, most will have become grandparents, the vast majority will have retired from work, and almost all will be planning to enjoy their remaining lifetime in as good general condition as possible.

However, when cancer knocks on the elderly door, it just comes as a truly catastrophic event, exactly as it happens in the youngest one; such bad news has indeed the weight to put life into jeopardy, while the perspective of dying is quite logically coming closer and closer.

Many cancers, though, become chronic conditions, and their management may require serious additional resources. These may be limited by personal or societal realities because the costs of treatments will also have to be taken into account. Ageism may intervene to disturb appropriate management since it is an attitude frequently observed in both lay people and health professionals. Inequity may thus be not so far as it has been well demonstrated by multiple studies showing that cancers have a worse prognosis in senior adults than in younger patients.

Very soon, the third and fourth ages will represent about 20% of the entire population in low-income countries to 30% in high-income countries. This calls for a rapid adaptation of our respective social and health systems to preserve intergeneration solidarity, thus raising questions such as the following:

- What space does society intend to leave to its most senior citizens?
- How should the elderlies behave to keep their position safe?
- Or, which roles do senior adults want to play in their future?
- When death approaches, is there a right time to die?

Medical oncologists are faced with the complexity of treating senior adults (elderly, older people) with cancer. If not lead and inspired by the Hippocrates oath, which appears nowadays sometimes not in keeping with the outside world reality, they should at least be lead and inspired by the concept of dignity that is attached to every human being on earth regardless of the subject's personal condition.

From the professional point of view, senior adults with cancer deserve the following (Fig. 1).

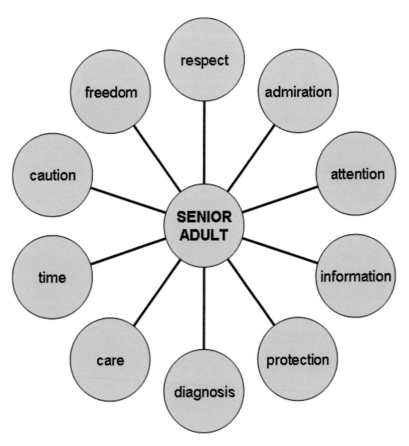

Figure 1 The ten commandments in the care of senior adults.

Respect

Over the years, senior adults have gained experience in life. In every society, they are most of the time at least recognized as wisdom holders. In addition, many continue to take community responsibilities despite being put off work.

The question of life expectancy slowly surges as an evidence to them since most of their time has already been lived. However, remaining lifetime is an individual matter that is influenced by the personal genetic background and the environmental hazards.

▶ Healthy octogenarians have more time to live than sick septuagenarians, and nonagenarians can enjoy an additional four-year life expectancy that will still be over one year at the age of 100.

Admiration

Beside the ability to reach a respectable age, senior adults actually succeed to escape premature end of life. Lifestyle and nutritional aspects of daily living thus match epidemiological projections showing that the annual probability of dying is kept below 10% until the age of 70 years. In other words, the risk of dying rises from 1 in 10,000 at the age of 10 years to 1 in 10 at the age of 70 years and almost 1 in 1 at the age of 100 years.

▶ Similar trends are observed throughout the world, suggesting a welcome global improvement of living conditions for the general population.

Attention

The prevalence of chronic conditions at an advanced age will continue to increase. Cancer patients will thus present with concomitant cardiovascular diseases in up to half cases and more metabolic conditions such as diabetes mellitus. Cognitive deficits are present in more than a quarter of senior adults after the age of 80 years, thus raising questions about comprehension and informed consent. Senior adults also accumulate general risk factors for mortality such as functional decline, delirium, falls, incontinence, and neglect.

▶ An interdisciplinary approach is an attractive efficient way to tackle the multiple problems routinely encountered in senior adults.

Information

Senior adults were educated several decades ago when DNA had not been described and wireless communications had not even been imagined. Today, they listen, although what is said does not always correspond to what is understood. This may sometimes lead to misunderstandings and unrealistic expectations. They read and surf the internet to learn that five-year breast cancer survival probability is over 80% regardless of age at diagnosis provided standard adequate treatment is offered. Of great interest, published surveys have shown that quality of life (QoL), though being an ill-defined concept in senior adults, is more important for them than survival length.

▶ Additional efforts to properly communicate good news as well as bad news may help to share an active partnership with senior adults.

Protection

In democracy, senior adults are voting citizens, and their influence on critical decisions is by no way to be minimized. The gray power is, therefore, a growing reality asking for more interest from politicians and the society itself. About half of the senior adults live on their own in the urban community, and the proportion increases with age. In parallel, there is a feminization of the oldest old because women have a definitive life expectancy advantage on men. And in many communities, only half or less of those with biological descendants can rely on help and assistance of a nearby living child.

Thus, advanced directives should be actively promoted by health professionals who must then obey their content and listen carefully to the therapeutic representative.

▶ Needs of senior adults are therefore becoming more and more specific to the societal transformation of their daily environment.

Diagnosis

Senior adults are prone to cancer, with over 2,000 new cases per 100,000 inhabitants per year. This is a ten times higher incidence in comparison with the population below the age of 65 years. Accurate diagnosis leading to further appropriate tests aiming at the best-designed treatment is the single way to maintain or improve the quality of the remaining time to live.

▶ Professional geriatric evaluation, together with scientific assessment of cancer cells by the pathologist and precise medical oncologic clinical staging, is mandatory.

Care

Too many different drugs are prescribed to senior adults because of their comorbidities. The risks of interactions and detrimental side effects are well known at all times during the management of cancers and of other diseases. Poor outcomes have been reported, including fatal events caused by standard drugs. In addition, unlicensed substances, sometimes of a very poor quality, are used by as much as 50% of cancer patients. Optimal care should therefore encompass the traditional aspect of "*bona fama*" and complementary medicines.

▶ Four fundamental ethic principles must govern medical action with the aim to find a valid balance between each of them, which are the following (Fig. 2):

- *Autonomy* means the capacity to decide what is good or not good for one self; senior adults should fully understand the problematic before giving consent to further tests or therapeutic measures.
- *Justice (equity)* is the capacity for a group to distribute wealth on an equal basis and above all for the most in need; senior adults should benefit from the resources generated within a community to maintain and/or improve health conditions.
- *Beneficiency* is the capacity to do what is good for the other and of sanitary benefit; health professionals should use their skills to maintain and/or improve health conditions of senior adults.
- *Nonmaleficiency* is the capacity to not harm the other; health professionals should take every precaution to make sure that health conditions of senior adults are not at risk to be damaged by diagnostic or therapeutic measures.

Time

As is the case with children in pediatrics, senior adults are most of the time accompanied by loved ones. But these may not be members of their family. The traditional composition of families has indeed suffered many changes

Autonomy

Justice (equity)

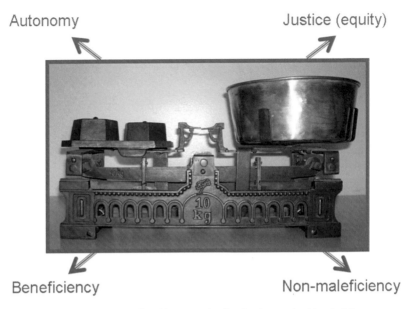

Beneficiency

Non-maleficiency

Figure 2 *The balance to be found between the four fundamental ethic principles.*

during the past century in relation with the observed increased life expectancy. In many countries, a high incidence of divorce has profoundly modified intrafamilial communication and composition. Senior adults and proxies may thus require more time for explanations and understanding of their personal situation. Distance to and from health centers may hamper access to care requiring transport facilitation to be organized and social intervention to be implemented.

▶ Family and/or the most significant proxy should not be left without help and assistance to minimize the risk of burnout.

Caution

Senior adults use vulnerable and frail organs with a progressive reduction of the tolerance to stress and a loss of functional reserves. Striated muscles are replaced by increased fat, kidney function loses as much as 1 mL/min/yr from the age of 40 years, and liver function is not as efficient at 80 years as it was at 50. But the worrying limitation is the incidence of cognitive troubles and the occurrence of dementia, which markedly increase with age to reach unexpected levels.

▶ Short assessment will provide useful information but will not preclude a more thorough neuropsychological evaluation to ascertain harmlessness.

Freedom

Thoughts and beliefs are daily life companions allowing the development of a personal spirituality. In many senior adults, the persistence or the resurgence of religious feelings must receive an appropriate answer. To cope with cancer, senior adults tend indeed to use prayers first before music, exercise, or meditation. On the other hand, in a few countries around the world, assisted suicide and/or euthanasia are now integrated in medical practice and are supported by the population. Beside palliative care, this is the end chosen by a minority of senior adults when facing physical or psychological suffering from cancer diseases. None of this should be ignored.

Please remember that historians judge the degree achieved by successful civilizations through the way they care for the weakest, the poorest, and the oldest.

Declaration of Interest:
Dr Zulian has not reported any conflicts of interest.

Further Reading

Chochinov HM. Dignity and the essence of medicine: the A, B, C and D of dignity conserving care. BMJ 2007; 335:184–187.

Fallowfield L, Jenkins V. Current concepts of communication skills training in oncology. Recent Results Cancer Res 2006; 168:105–112.

Kearney N, Miller M. Elderly patients with cancer: an ethical dilemma. Crit Rev Oncol Hematol 2000; 33:149–154.

Walter LC, Covinsky KE. Cancer screening in elderly patients: a framework for individualized decision making. JAMA 2001; 285:2750–2756.

The Role of the Multidisciplinary Team

L. Balducci

H. Lee Moffitt Cancer Center and Research Institute, Tampa, Florida, U.S.A.

Introduction

The management of cancer is multidisciplinary virtually all times, as it involves different oncologic specialties. In the case of the older-aged person, the scope of the multidisciplinary team encompasses areas outside cancer and even outside the medical domains.

As comorbidity is a hallmark of age, the team includes professionals experienced in the management of diseases other than cancer. The intervention of other professionals such as pharmacists, social workers, and dieticians is also required to make treatment accessible, safe, and effective. Last but not least, the role of the nurse is pivotal in the management of older cancer patients. By training, the nurse—who in German is called "Krankenschwester," sister of the sick—is focused on the welfare of the whole person. Striking the ideal balance of medical and personal needs in each individual situation is the nurse's unique expertise. In addition, the nurse is attuned to vocalize the patient's unspoken needs and to identify early signs of discomfort and decompensation and to bring them to the attention of the proper professional.

Aging involves a progressive reduction in the functional reserve of multiple organs and systems and increased prevalence of comorbidity. This results in a reduction of a person's life expectancy and stress tolerance and increases the risk of disability and functional dependence. In the meantime, cognitive restrictions and socioeconomic limitation may lessen the ability of the older person to compensate for his or her functional losses. Depression, malnutrition, and polypharmacy may further enhance the vulnerability and the disability of the aged.

The goals of cancer treatment in the older-aged person include prolongation of active life expectancy (that may also be referred to as compression of morbidity), in addition to the traditional goals of cure, prolongation of survival, maintenance of quality of life, and symptom management.

The management of the older person with or without cancer has to include multiple and different needs that imply a return to a brand of holistic medicine all but forgotten at the times of specialized fast food–inspired medicine. This is the medicine practiced in highly specialized centers, such as anticancer, cardiologic, or orthopedic centers that offer only services limited to that specialty. The "we do this one food right" type of medicine is rarely beneficial to the older-aged person, who may die of a heart attack or become disabled while receiving "state-of-the-art" treatment for prostate or breast cancer. The team approach to the older cancer patients thus involves more than the welfare of the individual patient. It is a proposition and a demonstration of a medicine attuned to the aging of the population.

In this chapter, we will provide three examples of the multidisciplinary approach to the older cancer patients in three critical areas: geriatric assessment, management of polypharmacy, and caregiver support. We will conclude with an overview of the team function and of future perspectives.

The Assessment of Age

The basic questions of geriatric oncology include the patient's life expectancy and treatment tolerance.

- So far, the best-validated estimate of life expectancy has been obtained by integrating comorbidity and function (Fig. 1). Lee et al. have given a score to age, specific functions, and comorbidities in home-dwelling individuals 70 years and older and have been able to predict accurately the risk of four-year mortality. This model is being continuously refined to be applied to both ambulatory and hospitalized individuals.
- The comprehensive geriatric assessment (CGA) also provides an estimate of the risk of chemotherapy-related hematological and non-hematological toxicity. It has been known for several years that instrumental activity of daily living (IADL) dependence was an indicator for complications from cytotoxic chemotherapy. A recent study that is being currently analyzed has involved more than 500 patients

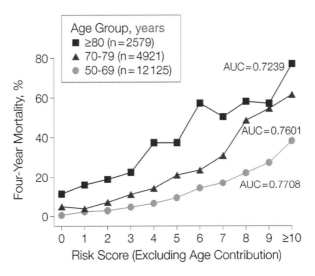

Figure 1 *Estimate of four-year mortality for patients aged 70 and older on the basis of function and comorbidity. Abbreviation: AUC: area under the curve. Source: From Lee et al.*

70 years and older integrated 25 parameters in the prediction of chemotherapy complications (Exterman M, Druta M, Popa M. Personal communication, AACR, Denver Colorado, 2009). The chemotherapy risk assessment scale in high-age patients (CRASH) score will represent the frame of reference for further studies of this subject and for planning the treatment of older cancer patients.

Other benefits of the CGA involve recognition of conditions that may interfere with cancer treatment, such as cognitive disorders, depression, especially subclinical depression, nutritional risk, polypharmacy, and absence of an adequate caregiver. Some of these conditions may be reversible, and others may be compensated for with proper intervention. For example, a patient with memory disorders may require the assignment of a caregiver prior to the start of chemotherapy; a patient unable to use transportation may need the designation of a driver.

While there is general agreement that a CGA is essential to the management of older cancer patients, controversy lingers over its execution. Several practices have adopted some form of screening test to identify patients who need a more "in-depth" assessment. In any case, the CGA implies a multidisciplinary team. While the initial evaluation of the patient, including functional assessment, is best performed by a nurse, a social worker is needed for assessing cognition, living conditions, and availability of a caregiver, a pharmacist for the assessment of polypharmacy, and a nutritionist for the assessment of nutrition and nutritional risk. Ideally, the team should also have access to other medical specialists including cardiologists, neurologists, endocrinologists, and nephrologists; to a minister of the appropriate faith trained for the recognition and management of spiritual and existential distress; and to a physical therapist.

The role of the team in the CGA is not limited to the estimate of functional age. It also involves the management of conditions that may compromise cancer treatment and may lead to functional dependence. This task will be described in the team function.

Polypharmacy

The prevalence of polypharmacy increases with age because, in part, of increased prevalence of comorbidity and, in part, of the increased utilization of over-the-counter medications and of alternative medicine products by older individuals.

A definition of polypharmacy is wanted, but a number of issues are clear.

- Cancer patients 70 years and older take an average of 11 non-cancer-related medications per patient.
- The risk of drug interactions increases geometrically for patients taking more than five medications on a single day.
- For patients taking eight medications each day, the risk of drug interaction is almost certain.
- Polypharmacy is a major cause of iatrogenic morbidity and mortality.

In a study performed at our institution, the interaction between cancer-unrelated drugs was associated with an 80% increase in the risk of chemotherapy complications.

Several studies in elderly patients with and without cancer have shown that polypharmacy is best managed when a pharmacist is part of the treatment team. In this the pharmacist may be helped by a computer program capable of identifing all potential drug interactions and by a number of criteria

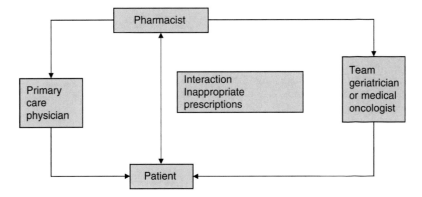

Figure 2 The pharmacist is central to identify inappropriate prescriptions. This information may be conveyed to the geriatrician or the oncologist on the team or to the patient's primary physician.

describing inappropriate prescriptions in the elderly. In addition to medication interactions, these include utilization of medications that are partially contraindicated in older age such as benzodiazepines or nonsteroidal anti-inflammatory agents.

To estimate both risks and benefits of polypharmacy, it would be very helpful to have a physician with geriatric experience on the team. This is the case in some countries such as France where an ongoing cooperation of geriatricians and oncologists assures the safest and most effective treatment of older cancer patients. Alternatively, one should make sure that the older cancer patient may rely on a primary care physician to whom the team pharmacist should communicate all planned treatment changes. These alternative approaches are illustrated in Figure 2.

Management of the Caregiver

The home caregiver is essential to the management of older cancer patients, not only of those suffering from disability or memory disorders. The most basic requirement of the caregiver is to be readily available in case of emergency and to be capable of providing timely transportation of the patient to a care center. Ideally, the caregiver should be able to provide emotional support to the patient to enhance the adhesion to the treatment program; to assure that the patient receives adequate nutrition and exercise; and to identify signs of distress or deconditioning. The caregiver may function as the spokesperson of the family when many different family members are involved in the care of the patient and be required to mediate the conflicts among different relatives with different agendas.

As the caregiver has this central role in the management of the older cancer patient, the physician, with the help of the team, should be able to identify and support the caregiver.

The evaluation of the caregiver includes the identification of this person that is generally designed by the patient and to recognize potential shortcoming of the caregiver. Common problems include the following:

- The caregiver is an older spouse with health problems of his or her own. This person may not be able to undergo the heavy caregiving task and needs to be aided by a younger and healthier person. In extreme circumstances, when a more able caregiver is not found, the patient may need institutionalization at least for the treatment duration.
- The caregiver is an adult child, most commonly a daughter, with a profession and a family of her/his own. The main difficulty of this person is to accommodate in a busy schedule the demands of caregiving, those of the profession and of the younger family. This syndrome is referred to as the "Aeneas syndrome" from the Rafaello depiction of Aeneas in the "Vatican stanze." There the Trojan hero is represented as carrying his older father on his shoulder and holding his young son with his left hand. In this case, it is important to know if the caregiver can get adequate respite from other family members and can conciliate family and work.

Caregiving is associated with a number of health problems, at least in the case of caregiving for Alzheimer patients. These include increased mortality, increased incidence of depression, increased risk of repeated infections, and delayed wound healings.

The management of the caregiver is a responsibility of the whole team and includes the following:

- Provision of adequate information related to the patient health and the caregiver's own health risk, as well as health maintenance recommendations

- Instruction on how to address common problems of cancer treatment, such as nausea and vomiting, fever, delirium as well as depression and anger
- Instruction on the management of family conflicts
- Help in dealing with work-related and economic issues

The identification of the caregiver is generally a combined task for the nurse and the social worker. Being on the forefront of the patient's assessment, the nurse is in the best position to recognize the person on whom the patient can rely most for support. In parallel, the social worker has the competence to recognize the assets and liabilities of the designed caregiver and to negotiate adequate solutions for the patient's needs.

Correction of the caregiver's shortcomings (e.g., finding a younger and independent person to aid an elderly and disabled caregiver) is the responsibility of the social workers.

The training of the caregiver is a combined task of the team. The physician and nurse are responsible for instructing the caregiver on how to manage common problems that may occur during cancer treatment; the social worker has the central task to guide the caregiver to the maintenance of her/his own health and to work out social issues such as leave from work and help in children care; the dietitian illustrates the most effective techniques to maintain the patient's nutritional status; while the pharmacist is of assistance in assuring adherence to the treatment regimen and in minimizing the potential complications of drugs.

All team members are responsible to praise the caregiver and highlight the importance of caregiving. If the caregiver relies on faith for strength, the intervention of a minister may also be desirable.

Function of the Team

The organization of the team is not codified. In our institution, the H. Lee Moffitt Cancer Center, a geriatric team has been operating for 16 years. Though it has undergone some evolution, the basic organization has remained the same (Fig. 3). All cancer patients aged 70 years and older are screened by a nurse for age-related problems. Patients who screen positive undergo a consultation by the whole team that reports the finding to the physician who is responsible for the initial treatment plans.

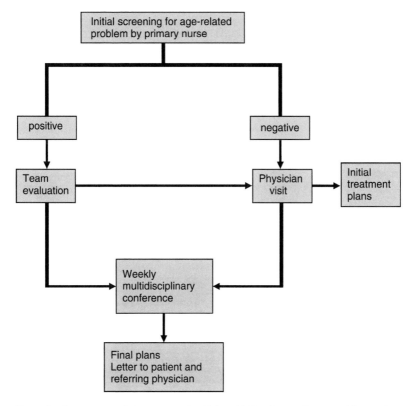

Figure 3 Organization of the team at the H. Lee Moffitt Cancer Center and Research Institute in Tampa.

All patients are discussed at the weekly multidisciplinary conference attended by the full team that issues final recommendations and a letter to the patient and the referring physician. During this informal discussion, new consultations are generated that might have been originally overlooked and all team members become aware of their own specific role in the management of the individual patient.

Of course, the function of the team is predicated on its cohesiveness and mutual trust of its members. Team building and team maintenance involve friendship, confidence, and open communication that are promoted by the team leader. This is not necessarily a physician; rather, the team professional who is more experienced in team building. The nurse practitioner and social worker have, at times, assumed such a role at our center.

Conclusions and Perspectives

The management of the older person with or without cancer implies a return to a patient-centered practice. This is best conducted by a multidisciplinary team, as a single person cannot manage any more the available wealth of information.

The delivery of care by a multidisciplinary team is one of the most important future research issues.

Declaration of Interest:
Dr Balducci has reported no conflicts of interest.

Further Reading

Balducci L, Cohen HJ, Engstrom Pf, et al. Senior adult oncology clinical practice guidelines in oncology. J Natl Compr Netw 2005; 3:572–590.

Carey EC, Covinsky KE, Lui LY, et al. Prediction of mortality in community-living frail elderly people with long-term care needs. J Am Geriatr Soc 2008; 56:68–75.

Dominguez LJ. Medicine and the Arts. L'incendio di Borgo. Commentary. Acad Med 2009; 84:1260–1261.

Extermann M, Hurria A. Comprehensive geriatric assessment in older patients with cancer. J Clin Oncol 2007; 25:1824–1831.

Hastings SN, Schmader KE, Sloane RJ, et al. Quality of pharmacotherapy and outcomes for older veterans discharged from the emergency department. J Am Geriatr Soc 2008; 56(5):875–880.

Lee SJ, Lindquist K, Segal MR, et al. Development and validation of a prognostic index for 4-year mortality in older adults. JAMA 2006; 295(7): 801–808.

Manton KG, Gu X, Lowrimore GR. Cohort changes in active life expectancy in the U.S. elderly population: experience from the 1982–2004 National Long-Term Care Survey. J Gerontol B Psychol Sci Soc Sci 2008; 63(5):S269–S281.

Ryan C, O'Mahony D, Byrne S. Application of STOPP and START criteria: interrater reliability among pharmacists. Ann Pharmacother 2009; 43(7):1239–1244.

Index

Aromatic amines
  bladder cancer and, 121
ASA. *See* American Society of
      Anesthesiologists (ASA)
Aspirin, 79
Assisted suicide, in medical practice, 171
ATAC trial
  tamoxifen, 47
ATG. *See* Antithymocyte globulin (ATG)
Attention, 167
Autonomy, ethic principles, 169
AZA. *See* 5-azacytidine (AZA)
5-Azacytidine (AZA), 89

B

Bacillus Calmette Guerin (BCG), 124
BC. *See* Bladder cancer (BC)
B-cell lymphoma, 68, 69
BCG. *See* Bacillus Calmette Guerin (BCG)
Beneficiency, ethic principles, 169
Benzodiazepines, 6, 163
  in older age, 176
Bevacizumab, 64, 142, 150
  for advanced non–small cell lung
      cancer, 105
  for breast cancer, 96
  for CRC, 112
BFI. *See* Brief fatigue inventory (BFI)
Bicalutamide, 52
BIG 1–98 study, 47
Bilateral salping-oophorectomy
  uterine cancer and, 132
Biological age, 1
Bisphosphonates, for metastatic breast
      cancer, 97
Black box warning, 159
Bladder cancer (BC), 121–127
  follow-up schedule of, 127
  history of, 122
  incidence of, 121
  mortality, 121
  organ-sparing treatments for, 126
  pathology, 121
  prognosis of, 126–127
  relative risk of developing, in smokers, 121

[Bladder cancer (BC)]
  risk factors for, 121
  signs and symptoms of, 122
  staging of, 123–124
  treatment of
    radical radiotherapy for, 125
    surgical, 124–125
    TURB for, 124
  ultrasonography and, 122
  urinary cytopathology and, 123
Bone marrow biopsy, 66
Bone pain, 4
Brachytherapy
  for treatment of prostate cancer, 116
Breast cancer, 3
  CYP2D6 inhibitors in, 49
  early stage of
    adjuvant chemotherapy for, 93–94
    adjuvant endocrine treatment for, 93
    primary hormonal therapy for, 92
    radiotherapy for, 93
    surgical approach in, 92
    trastuzumab for, 95
  hormonal agents, 46
  locally advanced, 95
  metastatic
    biological agents for, 96
    bisphosphonates for, 97
    chemotherapy for, 95–96
    endocrine therapy for, 95
    (neo)adjuvant hormonal therapy, 46–49
    side effects of hormonal therapy in,
        50, 51
Brief fatigue inventory (BFI), 31
Bupropion, 160
Buserelin, 52
Buspirone, 164

C

Cancer
  demographics, 9–11
  impact of frailty, 25–27
  mortality rate, 10
  symptoms of, 4
  types of, 3

E

EAU. *See* European Association of Urology (EAU)
ED, SCLC. *See* Extensive-disease (ED), SCLC
EGFR. *See* Epidermal growth factor receptor (EGFR)
Elderly
 defined, 1
 frailty in, 22–25
ELN. *See* European LeukemiaNet (ELN) guidelines
EMEA. *See* European Medicinal Agency (EMEA)
EMRT. *See* External megavoltage radiotherapy (EMRT)
Endocrine therapy
 for breast cancer, 93, 95
Endogenous erythropoietin (EPO), 86
Endometrial stromal sarcomas
 treatment of, 134, 135
EORTC. *See* European Organization for Research and Treatment of Cancer (EORTC)
Epidermal growth factor receptor (EGFR), 146
Epigenetic therapies
 for MDS, 89–90
Epirubicin, 107
EPO. *See* Endogenous erythropoietin (EPO)
ER. *See* Estrogen receptor (ER)
Erlotinib
 for advanced non–small cell lung cancer, 105
Erythropoiesis, 79
Erythropoiesis-stimulating agents (ESA), 67, 86
 nordic score to predict MDS, 87
ESA. *See* Erythropoiesis-stimulating agents (ESA)
Essential thrombocythemia (ET), 72
Estrogen
 for metastatic prostate cancer, 55
Estrogen receptor (ER), 46
ET. *See* Essential thrombocythemia (ET)

Etoposide, 107
EU. *See* European Union (EU)
European Association of Urology (EAU), 114
European EORTC trials
 with pelvic tumors, 41
European LeukemiaNet (ELN) guidelines, 76
European Medicinal Agency (EMEA), 88
European Organization for Research and Treatment of Cancer (EORTC), 37
 database of, 38
European Union (EU), 151
Euthanasia, in medical practice, 171
Everolimus, 150, 151
Extensive-disease (ED), SCLC, 106
External megavoltage radiotherapy (EMRT), 39

F

FAB. *See* French-American-British (FAB)
Fallopian tube cancer, 139, 141
 staging of, 141
Falls, 6–7
Fatigue, renal cell carcinoma, 148
FDA. *See* Food and Drug Agency (FDA)
Febrile neutropenia, 94
Fédération Internationale de Gynécologie Obstétrique (FIGO) staging system
 for cervical cancer, 128–131
 for Fallopian tube cancer, 141
 for ovarian cancer, 140
 for uterine cancer, 132–133
 for vaginal cancer, 134, 136
FIGO staging system. *See* Fédération Internationale de Gynécologie Obstétrique (FIGO) staging system
FISH. *See* Fluorescence in situ hybridization (FISH)
Fluorescence in situ hybridization (FISH), 76
5-fluorouracil (5FU), 110, 112
 leucovorin and, 110
Flutamide, 52
FOLFOX, 110, 112
Follow-up schedule, of bladder cancer, 127
Food and Drug Agency (FDA), 88

I

IADL. *See* Instrumental activity of daily
living (IADL)
IFN therapy. *See* Interferon (IFN) therapy
IL-6. *See* Interleukin (IL)-6
Imatinib
in CML, 76
efficacy of, 76
toxicity of, 76
IMiD. *See* Immunomodulating drug
(IMiD)
Immune thrombocytopenic purpura
(ITP), 88
Immunomodulating drug (IMiD), 88
IMRT. *See* Intensity-modulated radiotherapy
(IMRT)
Information, 168
Insomnia
medication for, 163–164
Instrumental activity of daily living (IADL),
15, 27
Intensity-modulated radiotherapy (IMRT), 39
Intensive therapies
for MDS, 90
Interferon-α, 78
Interferon (IFN) therapy
for mRCC, 150
Interleukin (IL)-6, 25
Intermittent androgen blockade
for advanced prostate cancer, 54
International prognostic index (IPI), 66
International Prognostic Scoring System
(IPSS), 83
risk score of, 84
International Society of Geriatric Oncology
(SIOG), 95
Prostate Cancer Task Force, 115
conclusion, 117
Interpersonal therapy (IPT), 161
Intravenous pyelogram (IVP)
bladder cancer and, 122–123
IPI. *See* International prognostic index (IPI)
IPSS. *See* International Prognostic Scoring
System (IPSS)
IPT. *See* Interpersonal therapy (IPT)

Irinotecan, 111
Iron chelation, 86–88
ITP. *See* Immune thrombocytopenic purpura
(ITP)
IVP. *See* Intravenous pyelogram (IVP)

J

Justice (equity), ethic principles, 169

K

Ketoconazole, 52
for metastatic prostate cancer, 55
Krankenschwester, 172

L

Lapatinib, 96
LD, SCLC. *See* Limited-disease (LD), SCLC
LDH. *See* Serum lactate dehydrogenase
(LDH)
Leiomyosarcomas
treatment of, 134, 135
Lenalidomide, 88
Letrozole, 96
Leucovorin (LV)
5FU and, 110
Lewy body disease, 6
LHRHa. *See* Luteinizing hormone-releasing
hormone agonists (LHRHa)
Life expectancy, by comorbidity and
function, 173
Lifestyle, probability of death and, 167
Limited-disease (LD), SCLC, 106
Liposomal doxorubicin, 96
LiverMetSurvey registry, 112
Lung cancer, 3, 98–107
NSCLC. *See* Non–small cell lung cancer
(NSCLC)
palliative radiotherapy for, 107
SCLC. *See* Small cell lung cancer (SCLC)
Luteinizing hormone-releasing hormone
agonists (LHRHa), 117
LV. *See* Leucovorin (LV)
LVSI. *See* Lymphovascular space invasion
(LVSI)

Lymphoma
  assess therapeutic options in, 69
  diagnosis of, 66–68
  overview, 66
  prognosis of, 66–68
  treatment of, 68–70
Lymphovascular space invasion (LVSI), 129

M

MACH-NC. *See* Meta-Analyses of
    Chemotherapy in Head and Neck
    Cancer (MACH-NC)
Mammalian target of rapamycin
    (mTOR), 150
MAOI. *See* Monamine oxidase inhibitor
    (MAOI)
MDS. *See* Myelodysplastic syndromes (MDS)
MDV 3100, 52, 55
Medical action, ethic principles for, 169
Medicare database, 110
Mental disorders
  anxiety, 161–164
  depression, 157–161
Meta-Analyses of Chemotherapy in Head
    and Neck Cancer (MACH-NC), 145
Metastatic breast cancer
  biological agents for, 96
  bisphosphonates for, 97
  chemotherapy for, 95–96
  endocrine therapy for, 95
Metastatic prostate cancer, 55
Metastatic renal cell carcinoma (mRCC)
  medical management of, 149–153
  phase III clinical trials, summary of, 151
Methicillin-resistant *Staphylococcus aureus*
    (MRSA) infection, 34
MGA. *See* Multidimensional geriatric
    assessment (MGA)
MIBC. *See* Muscle-invasive bladder cancer
    (MIBC)
Mini-mental status (MMS) examination, 15
Mirtazapine, 159, 160
MMS. *See* Mini-mental status (MMS)
    examination
Monamine oxidase inhibitor (MAOI), 159

Monotherapy, with GnRH agonist
  for advanced prostate cancer, 54
MOSAIC trial, 110
mRCC. *See* Metastatic renal cell carcinoma
    (mRCC)
mTOR. *See* Mammalian target of rapamycin
    (mTOR)
Mucosal reactions, 38
Mucositis, 60
Multidimensional geriatric assessment
    (MGA), 15
  packages for, 19–20
Multidisciplinary approach
  caregiver support, 176–178
  function, 178–180
  in geriatric assessment, 173–175
  in polypharmacy management, 175–176
Muscle-invasive bladder cancer (MIBC)
  systemic CT for, 126
Myelodysplastic syndromes (MDS)
  age-adjusted models, 85–86
  epigenetic therapies, 89–90
  growth factors for, 86–88
  immunomodulating agents, 88
  intensive therapies for, 90
  iron chelation, 86–88
  relevance of, 82
  transfusion therapy for, 86–88
Myeloproliferative disorders (MPD)
  classification of, 72–76
  CML, 76
  diagnosis of, 72–76
  imatinib in, 76–77
  polythemia vera, 77–78
  primary myelofibrosis, 79
Myelosuppression, 58

N

National Cancer Institute (NCI), 9
National Cancer Institute of Canada
    (NCIC), 100
National Comprehensive Cancer Network
    (NCCN), 118, 154
National Surgical Adjuvant Breast and
    Bowel Project (NSABP), 94

Printed and bound by CPI Group (UK) Ltd, Croydon, CR0 4YY

23/10/2024

01777709-0001